Nursing - New Perspectives

Edited by Serpil Çelik Durmuş

Published in London, United Kingdom

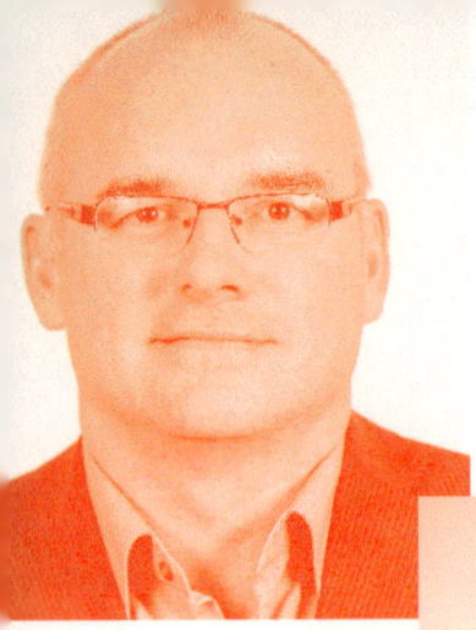
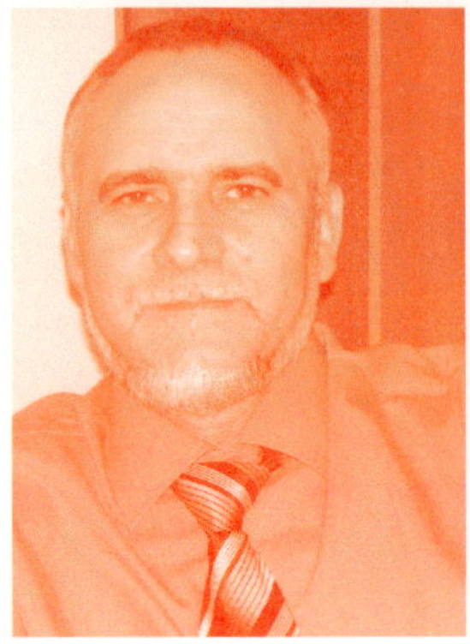
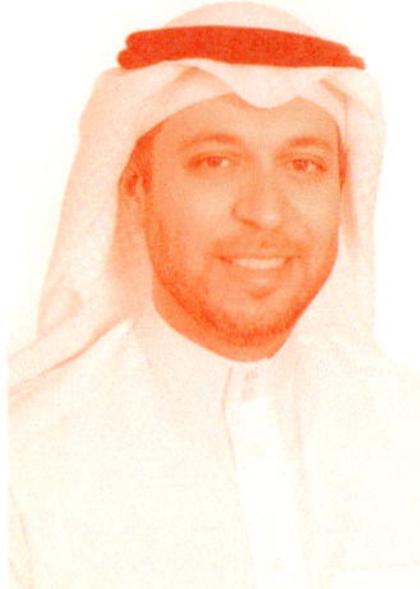
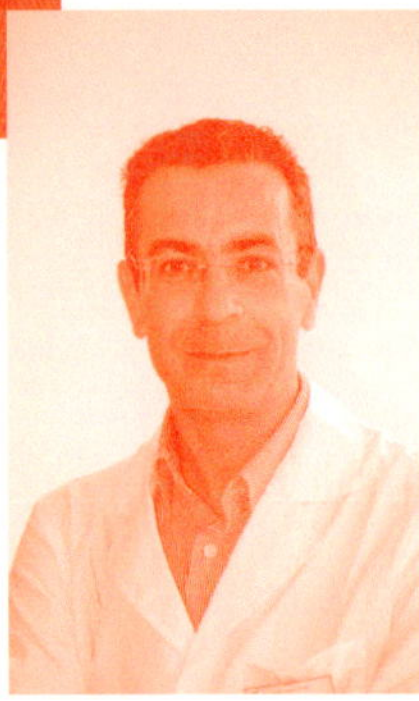
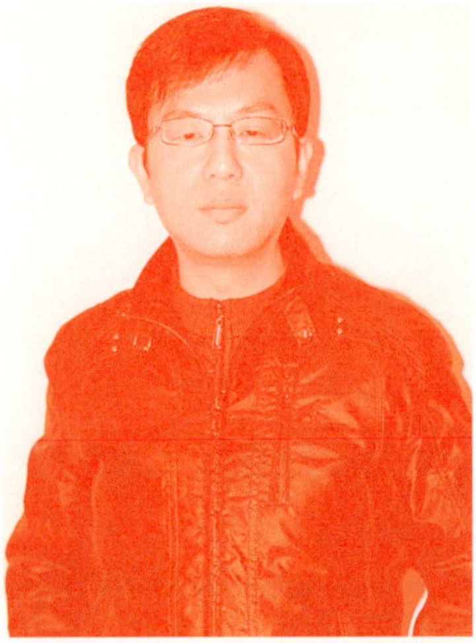
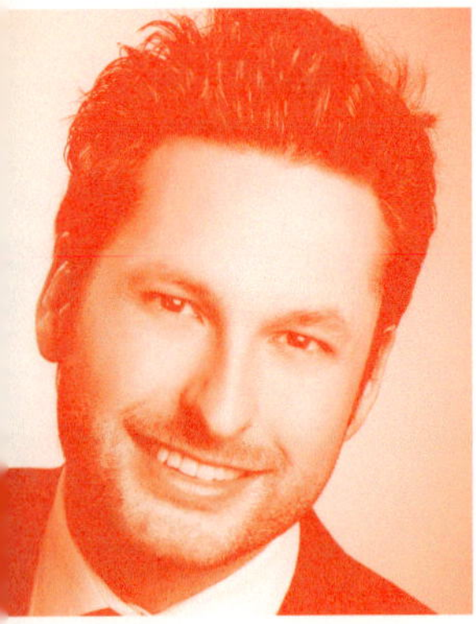
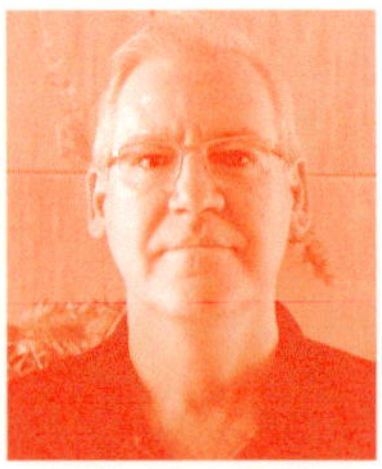

IntechOpen

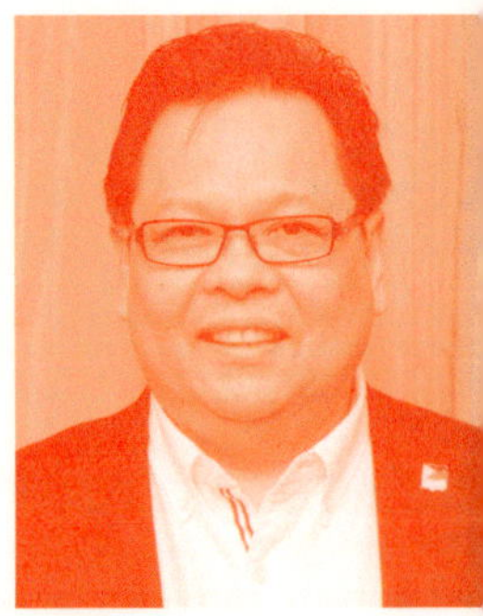
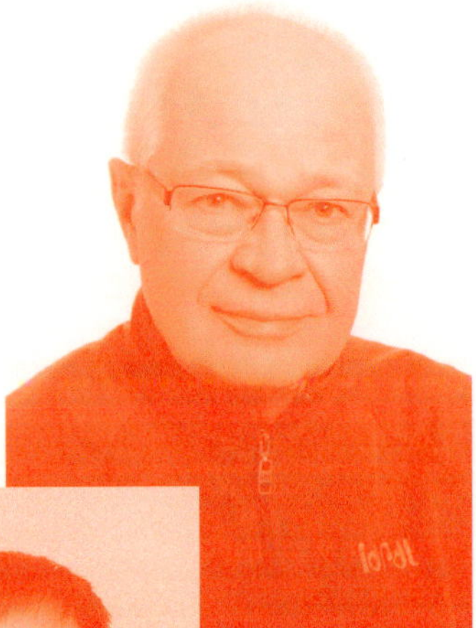
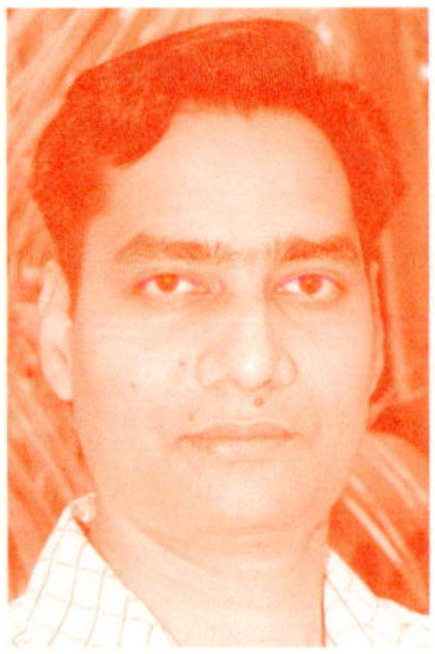
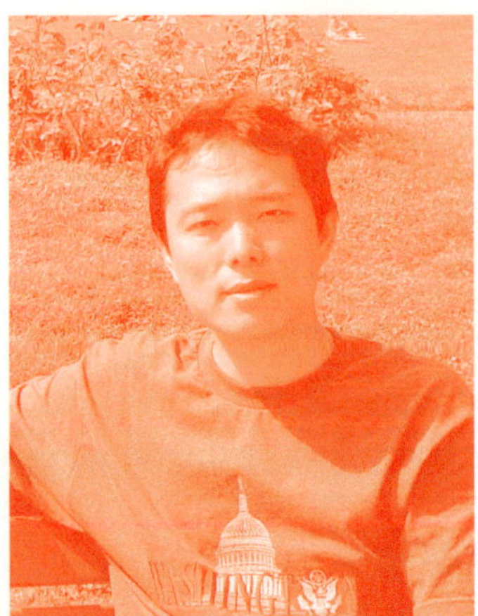
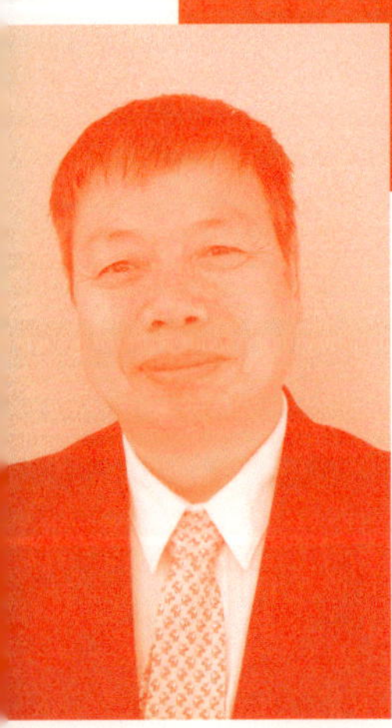
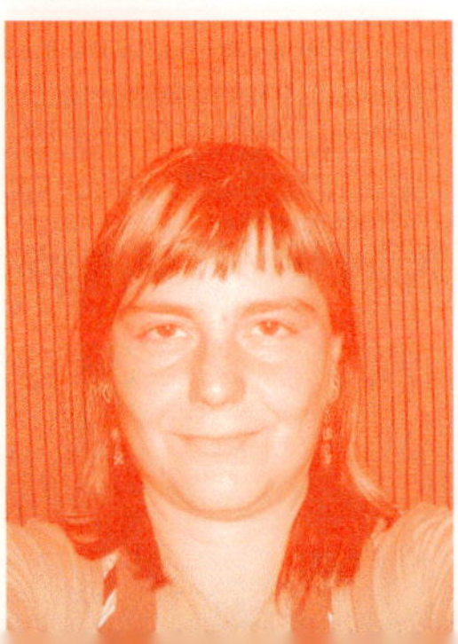

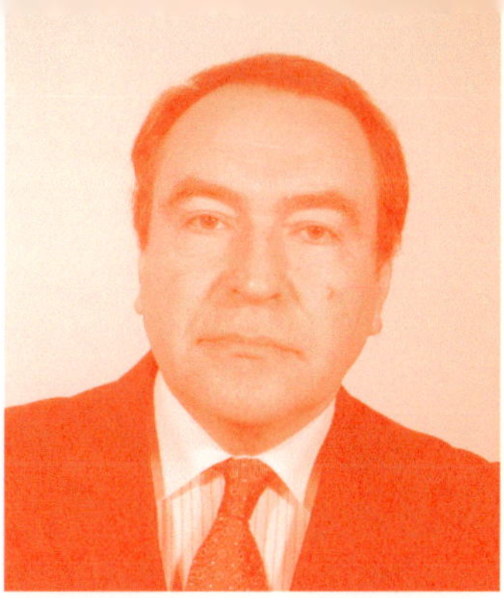
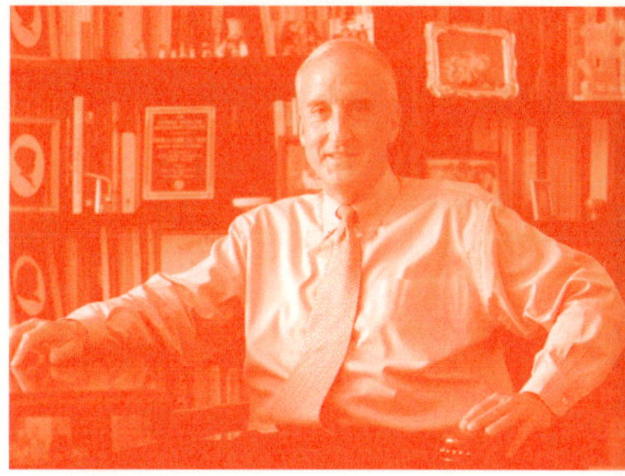
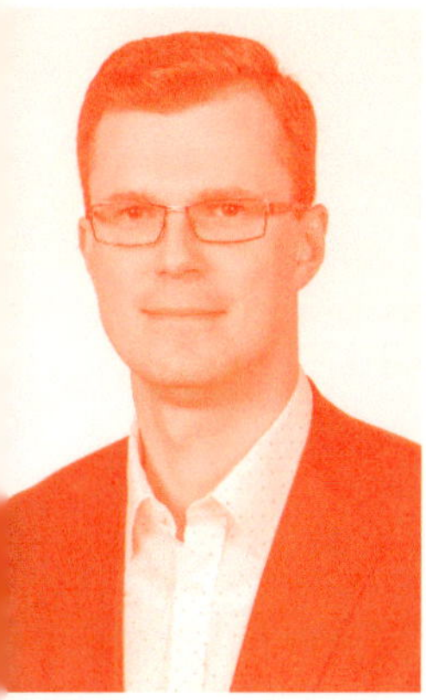
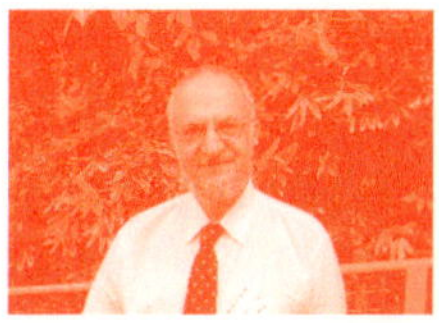
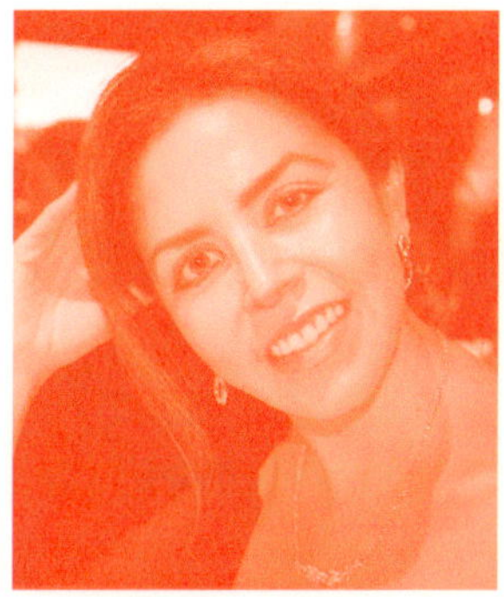

Supporting open minds since 2005

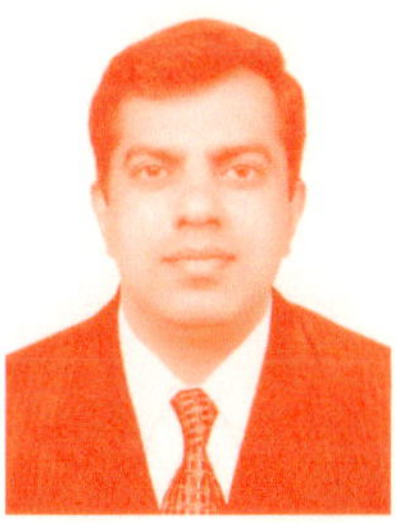
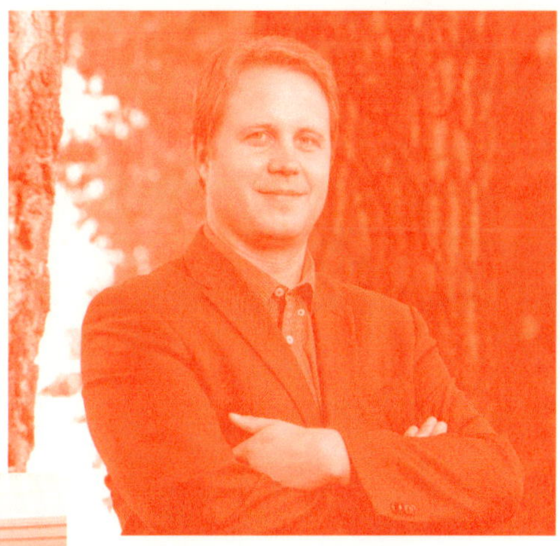
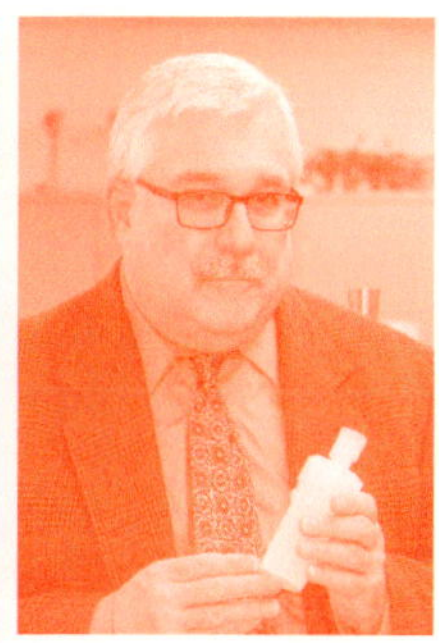
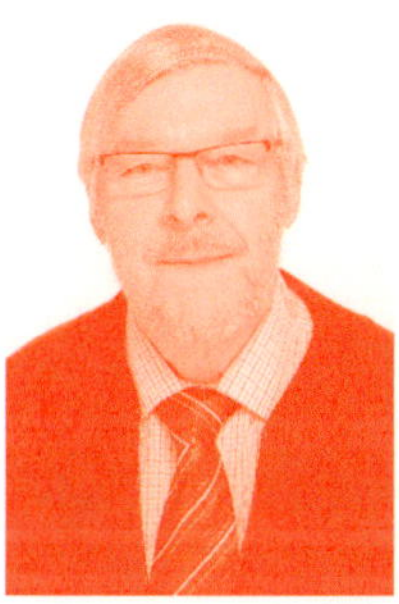
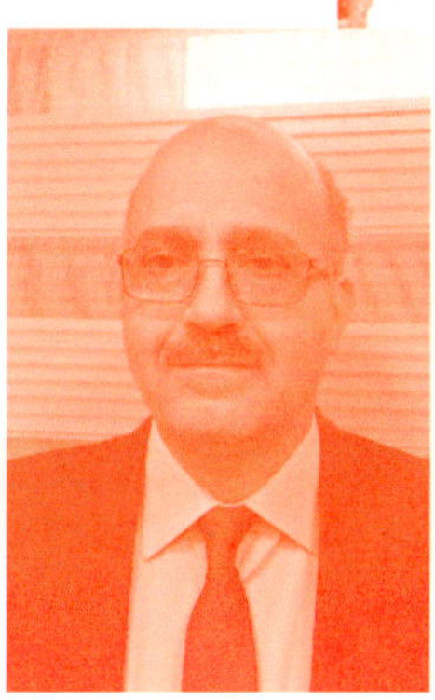
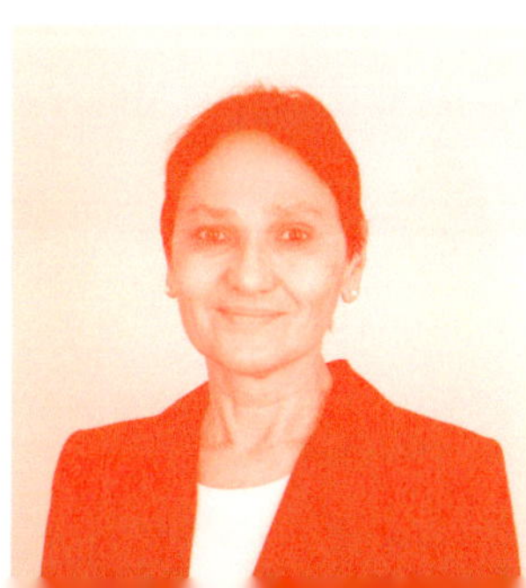
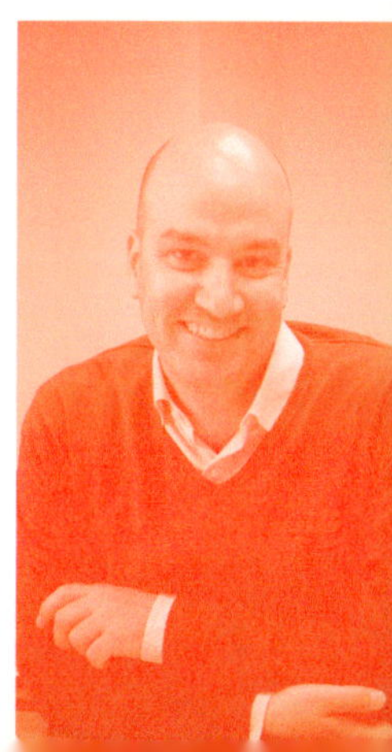

Nursing - New Perspectives
http://dx.doi.org/10.5772/intechopen.83042
Edited by Serpil Çelik Durmuş

Scientific Contributor: Jawahar (Jay) Kalra

Contributors
Eliana Escudero, Marlova Silva, Marcia Corvetto, Serpil Çelik Durmuş, Kamile Kirca, Natasha Khamisa, Carmen Luisa Betancur Pulgarín, Yudi Nathalia Angulo Ante, Yaqueline Churi Antero, Luis Gabriel Murillo Micolta, Mónica Roció Romero Carvajal, Mayumi Uno, Theresa Gaffney, Diego Carmona Carmona

First published in London, United Kingdom, 2021 by IntechOpen
IntechOpen is the global imprint of INTECHOPEN LIMITED, registered in England and Wales, registration number: 11086078, 5 Princes Gate Court, London, SW7 2QJ, United Kingdom
Printed in Croatia

British Library Cataloguing-in-Publication Data
A catalogue record for this book is available from the British Library

Additional hard and PDF copies can be obtained from orders@intechopen.com

Nursing - New Perspectives
Edited by Serpil Çelik Durmuş
p. cm.
Print ISBN 978-1-78985-971-3
Online ISBN 978-1-78985-972-0
eBook (PDF) ISBN 978-1-83962-929-7

For EU product safety concerns:
IN TECH d.o.o., Prolaz Marije Krucifikse Kozulić 3, 51000 Rijeka, Croatia, info@intechopen.com or visit our website at intechopen.com.

Meet the editor

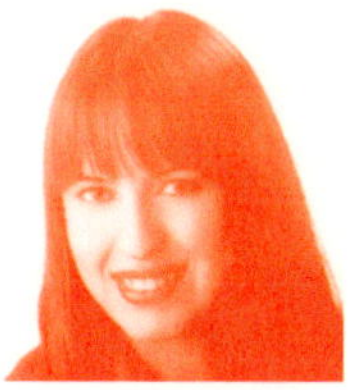

Serpil Çelik Durmu was born in 1985 in Nevşehir/Turkey. After graduating from Gazi University School of Nursing in 2007, she completed her master's degree at the same university in the Department of Nursing Management. Later, in 2015, she completed her doctorate at the Istanbul University Institute of Health Sciences, Department of Nursing Management. She worked as a research assistant at Düzce University and Istanbul University between 2009 and 2016. Since 2016, she has been working as an Assistant Professor at Kırıkkale University Faculty of Health Sciences, Department of Nursing. Her education is in the field of management in nursing and her areas of interest included quality in health, medical errors, professionalization in the profession, teamwork, patient safety, and ethical issues.

Contents

Preface

This book, Nursing New Perspectives, was written to make an important contribution to the field of nursing. Authors from all over the world have contributed to the book according to their areas of expertise and study topics. The book, which includes current and interesting topics such as nursing leadership, simulation and communication-collaboration, is an important acquisition for the nursing field.

I would like to thank all the authors and the IntechOpen family who contributed to the writing of the book.

Serpil Çelik Durmuş
Nursing Management Department,
Faculty of Health Sciences,
Kırıkkale University,
Kırıkkale, Turkey

Section 1

Nursing Leadership and Simulation

Chapter 1

Leadership Styles in Nursing

Serpil Çelik Durmuş and Kamile Kırca

Abstract

Recent developments in the field of management-organization and organizational behavior and new concepts have also led to the emergence of new leadership styles in leadership. Leadership in health services is important for following innovations and adapting to current situations. Nurses working together with other health personnel in hospitals providing health services constitute an important group in leadership. Nursing, which is a key force for patient safety and safe care, is a human-centered profession, and therefore leadership is a key skill for nurses at all levels. The leadership styles of nurse managers are believed to be an important determinant of job satisfaction and persistence of nurses. The need for nurses with leadership skills and the need for nurses to develop their leadership skills are increasing day by day. There are several leadership styles defined in nursing literature. These leadership styles are examined under the titles of relational leadership style, transformational leadership, resonant leadership, emotional intelligence leadership, and participatory leadership. The task-focused leadership style is explored under the headings of transactional and autocratic leadership, laissez-faire leadership, and instrumental leadership.

Keywords: nursing, leadership, leadership styles, patient safety, quality of care

1. Introduction

"Leadership is not only about individuals, but also about teams" [1].

Nowadays, leadership in health services is an important issue that aims to protect and improve human health. Rapid changes and developments in the health sector increase the importance of developing managership and leadership skills for health managers [2]. Regional and national health systems tend to redesign their functions and priorities by making structural changes in social and economic terms to cope with the increasing health problems [3]. The inclusion of complex technology and intense human relations in hospital services, which constitute a significant part of health care services, leads to the emergence of important managerial problems [4]. The existence of effective, creative, visionary, motivated, knowledgeable, principled leaders for the development of the institution is important to eliminate various problems in health services. To be able to do this, it is necessary to determine the qualifications that can contribute to the effective leadership of corporate managers [2, 5].

Leadership in health services is of great importance in terms of following innovations and adapting to existing situations [6]. Leadership can be defined as a multidimensional process, which means that a person motivates others to direct their activities and develop their skills under certain circumstances [3, 7]. The leader is the person who sets the goals of his group and who influences and directs the members of the group in line with these goals [8]. In addition, a good leader must be dynamic, passionate, have a motivational effect on other people, be solution oriented, and try to inspire others. Nurses, who work together with other health personnel in hospitals, constitute an important group in leadership. Nursing, which is a key force for patient safety and safe care, is a human-centered profession, and therefore leadership is a key skill for nurses at all levels. The leadership styles of nurse managers are believed to be an important determinant of job satisfaction and job commitment of nurses. Nurses who are mobilized and empowered to perform specific personal or group goals by a good leader nurse are willing to implement evidence-based practices and are highly motivated, well informed, and committed to organizational goals. Therefore, they perform patient care in a more effective and planned process. It has become imperative to examine the role of leadership styles of nurse managers on staff outcomes after miscarriage of health workforce, which is a global nursing problem, increasing health care costs and workload [9, 10].

There is a limited number of articles in the literature about the leadership styles of nurses. In these studies, the importance of leadership styles and practices on patient outcomes and patient safety, health service power and corporate culture were determined [3]. However, Cummings [10] stated that most styles can be grouped under relational leadership or task-focused leadership. Relational leadership styles focus on people and relationships. It includes transformational, emotional intelligence, resonance, and participatory leadership. These styles are positively associated with staff satisfaction, organizational commitment, improved staff health welfare, stress reduction, job satisfaction, productivity increase, effective study, and positive patient outcomes. However, task-focused leadership is focused on completion of works, deadlines, and directives. Task-focused leadership styles include operational, autocratic, and laissez-faire leadership [10].

2. Leadership styles in nursing

2.1 Relational leadership

Relational leadership styles focus on people and relationships and include transformational, emotional intelligence, resonance, and participatory leadership [11]. These leadership styles are associated with increased employee satisfaction, organizational commitment, improved staff health and well-being, stress reduction, job satisfaction, increased productivity, effective work, and positive patient outcomes [10].

2.1.1 Transformational leadership

Transformational leadership is considered the gold standard of leadership [11]. Transformational leadership is at the center of nursing because it has an impact on patient outcomes, employee satisfaction, and safety culture. Transformational nurse leaders first perform nursing, communicate effectively with their audiences, and become effective role models [12]. Such leaders are motivated and empowering, encouraging and following their audience for organizational goals and individual goals [13, 20]. In addition, it is explained how the transformational leaders have four characteristics that affect their audience. These characteristics are charisma, inspirational, intellectual thinking, and individual attention [42].

It is thought that the transformational leaders fascinate their audience with the charisma feature. This fascination is sometimes associated with the physical characteristics of the leader as well as communication skills and vision. The inspiring character of transformational leaders supports and motivates their followers with encouraging speeches in case of hard work and crises [14].

Transformational leaders, with their intellectual characteristics, encourage their followers to think innovatively and to think about how we can do it better. At the same time, these leaders do not prefer their followers to accept their thoughts as they are [14]. Finally, the transformational leaders, who are interested in their followers individually, advise them in line with their individual needs. In addition, leaders appreciate their followers within the team.

When considered with a general assessment, transformational leaders think that their followers should be evaluated individually and the needs and characteristics of the followers may change with the influence of the leader. Therefore, with the mentoring of the leader, the development of the followers increases at the same rate.

2.1.2 Resonance leadership

Resonance leadership is based on emotional intelligence and awareness, including being open and sensitive to judgment [15]. Resonance leaders have emotional intelligence features. These are self-awareness, self-management, social awareness, and relationship management [16]. According to these characteristics, resonance leaders are effective in managing and solving conflict, democratic, collaborative, and can find solutions to problems.

2.1.3 Emotional intelligence

Emotional intelligence was first described as a feature of transformational and resonant leadership in the 1980s. Leaders with emotional intelligence have four important structures: self-awareness, self-management, social awareness, and social skills. Emotionally intelligent leaders are sensitive to the well-being, emotions, and emotional health of themselves and their followers, and develop effective personal relationships while directing followers to common business goals. Emotionally intelligent leaders manage and reflect their emotions, making rational decisions to ensure teamwork and collaboration. Emotionally intelligent leaders are also effective in conflict resolution because they have the ability to see the situation from others' perspective and manage work stress [11].

2.1.4 Participatory leadership

In participatory leadership, the views of individuals and groups are taken into consideration. Knowledge, experience, skills, and innovation are of great importance in the decision-making process, with a wide range of expertise and participation in engagement. In 2016, WHO called for participatory leadership to replace hierarchical leadership models of health leadership, suggesting that inclusiveness and the involvement of various stakeholders would strengthen health services [17].

2.2 Task-focused leadership

The task-focused leadership style involves planning business activities, clarifying roles within a team or a group of people, as well as a set of objectives, and continuous monitoring of processes and performance. Task-focused leaders focus on completion of jobs, deadlines, and directives [10]. Task-focused leadership is significantly associated with high-level patient satisfaction [18].

2.2.1 Transactional and autocratic leadership

"Do it now!"

This concept, which is referred to as "transactional leadership" in English literature, is used as "interactionist," "operational," or "transactional" leadership in different sources. Transactional leadership is a leadership style that provides short-term goals and motivates viewers through the fulfillment of individual needs in exchange for high performance toward organizational goals [19]. Leaders in transactional leadership act as exchanges managers by exchanging followers who lead to improvement in production, and are interested in processes rather than shared values with forward-thinking ideas [18, 20].

Transactional leadership style emerges in two basic forms as "management with exceptions" and "conditional rewarding" [21, 22]. The form management with exceptions is divided into two as active and passive. The active leader monitors the performance of the team followers and intervenes to correct these errors when he/she detects errors. The passive leader expects the followers' mistakes to draw their attention before giving negative feedback or any warning [23]. In conditional rewarding, transactional leaders clearly explain to their followers what their duties are, how they will be made, and how they will be rewarded if the desired tasks are fulfilled satisfactorily [21, 24].

Transactional leaders are cultural carriers who maintain the existing order and act in line with traditions and past [25]. In crises where an explicit orientation is required, the transactional leadership approach is an effective style. Transactional leadership can be the best leadership style for the direction of critical events [18, 26]. This leadership style can be effective in emergency situations such as cardiac arrest, by enabling nurses to focus on the task as a whole on the patient [27].

In the literature, transactional leadership and transformational leadership are explained together and comparisons are made. Besides, unlike the transformational leadership, leaders who adopt an interactive approach want to maintain the same things instead of changing the future, and they are less concerned with the creative and innovative aspects and focus on concepts such as efficiency and quality [28]. Bass emphasizes the use of interactive leadership as a conditionally rewarding performance, especially among followers and leaders [29]. While transformational leadership results in a performance beyond expected, interactive leadership focuses on the expected results [30]. According to the transactional leadership, leadership is seen as a simple mutual exchange between leaders and followers based on economic or political reasons, while transformational leadership states that leaders and followers influence each other in order to achieve higher levels of motivation and morale [31].

Another type of transactional leadership is autocratic leadership. Autocratic leaders are defined as directives, controlling, power-oriented, and closed-minded. The leader describes the "what, when, why, and how" of the task. He/she emphasizes obedience, loyalty, and strict adherence to the rules. Followers do what the autocratic leader says [32]. The autocratic leadership style can be considered ideal in emergencies because he or she takes all decisions himself/herself, regardless of the views of the leading staff [3]. Because information is seen as power, critical information can be hidden from the team. Mistakes are not tolerated and individuals are accused rather than erroneous operations. Rewards are given for compliance, but disobedience is punished [18, 32]. In addition, autocratic leaders can create fear among staff and often make decisions without consulting the team [32]. These leaders motivate their subordinates by using their "legal powers," "rewarding powers," and "coercive forces." Autocratic leaders may not be welcome by their team, but this can be transformed into appreciation and devotion when the positive results of their leadership emerge. Although staff do not like autocratic leaders, they often work well on their orders [18, 32]. This leadership approach can be useful at the moment when it is necessary to make quick decisions or to mobilize uneducated and less-motivated followers in the short term by pressure and fear [6, 33, 34]. The positive aspect of this style is that it works perfectly in emergencies or chaotic situations with little time for discussion.

Schoel et al. found that very popular leaders were perceived as ineffective, while unpopular leaders could be perceived as effective [35]. According to the results of Uysal et al., the perception of the behavior of hospital managers as autocratic by followers decreases the productivity of the work [6], because autocratic leadership is perceived negatively by the followers; the reason is that the authoritarian attitude does not give the employee the right to speak, and that the awards and punishments are precise and clear.

2.2.2 Laissez-faire leadership

The style of leadership recognizing full freedom is also referred to as "laissez-faire" in the literature and is expressed as "let them do it." This kind of a leader advises the process by not participating in the process, encourages followers to generate ideas, offers suggestions when asked by followers, and declares opinions. [31]. Leadership that recognizes full freedom is a style in which the leader provides little or no orientation or control, and prefers a practical approach. Fully free leadership style includes a leader who does not decide, and acts without staffing or supervision [3]. The main task of the leader is to provide resources. Such leaders dissipate responsibilities and retreat and refrain from taking decisions [31]. The leader only gives his/her opinion when asked about his/her opinion on any subject, but this view is not binding on his/her followers [36].

Leadership that recognizes full freedom is an authoritative, task-focused leadership style, because it involves the regulation of tasks in times of crisis, so it shows reactive leadership. This style of leadership is often used by inexperienced leaders or those who are about to vacate their leadership positions, who prefer to give up their followers or others to change their positions, such as those who would like to give up their job [18]. The leader leaves the followers on their own. Followers do what they think is the best. Followers are trained to find the best solution to their problems. Whenever he/she sees it necessary, a person can form a group with whom he/she wants to solve problems, try new ideas, and make the decisions that he/she thinks are most appropriate for him/her [37, 38].

There are positive and negative aspects of the leadership style that gives full freedom. The first positive aspect of this leadership style is the determination and implementation of the goals, plans, and policies of employees or members of the organization, and it mobilizes the creativity of each member or employee [39]. The second positive aspect is that employees are motivated to train themselves and find the most appropriate solution to the problems. When the individual deems it necessary, he/she creates a group with the people he/she wants, solves the problems, tries new ideas, and reaches the most appropriate decisions [40]. The negative aspects of leadership, which gives full freedom, are the emergence of turmoil within the organization and the fact that everyone leads to the targets he/she wants and even toward opposing targets. Another disadvantage is the significant decrease in organizational success, independent of personal achievements.

Skogstad et al. state that the type of leadership recognizing full liberty reinforces the role conflict and role ambiguity experienced by the individual, and increases the conflicts with colleagues [40]. Hinkin et al. also state that leadership behaviors that recognize full liberty harm the punitive and rewarding roles of the leader and decrease leaders' effectiveness [41]. Chaudhry and Javed state that fully free leadership has no effect on the motivation of the followers compared to other types of leadership [42]. Şentürk et al. reveals that fully free leadership does not have a reinforcing effect on innovative behaviors but rather reduces it [31]. According to the results of Uysal et al., the perception of the behavior of hospital managers as autocratic by followers decreases the productivity of the work [6]. Because autocratic leadership is perceived negatively by the followers. The reason is that the authoritarian attitude does not give the employee the right to speak, and that the awards and punishments are precise and clear.

2.2.3 Instrumental leadership

Instrumental leadership focuses on choosing an appropriate strategy along with appropriate resources to achieve business goals, and it is vital for sustainable corporate performance [43, 44]. This leadership style is part of the spectrum of transformational and interactive leadership styles. Instrumental leaders can be effective managers because they ensure efficiency protection. Thus, jobs are completed in line with the resources, strategic vision, and time constraints of the health facility [45]. In current leadership approaches, the strategy and task-focused developmental functions of the leaders are not taken into account; however, strategy and task-focused functions, which are instrumental forms of leadership, are essential for organizations and followers to ensure sustainable performance. Instrumental leadership is based on neither ideals nor swap relationships. Instrumental leadership includes ensuring harmony between the organization and the environment, developing strategies, preparing task and strategy tables, using resources effectively, and providing performance feedback [44]. The most prominent feature of the instrumental leadership type is the determination of the subordinates' path by the leader [34]. The instrumental leader is mainly concerned with the timely completion of the work related to the desired goal; it focuses on functions such as setting goals, organizing group members, setting up the communication system, and determining work-related times [46]. Akyurt et al. found that instrumental and interactive leadership have a statistically significant and positive effect on job satisfaction and organizational commitment [21]. Tengilimoglu and Yigit, in their study on 355 state hospital workers in order to determine the effect of leadership behavior in hospitals on job satisfaction of the employees, found that the leadership style with the highest job satisfaction were participatory, instrumental, success-oriented, and supporting leadership, respectively [34].

3. Effective leadership

As the health sector is in a process of change, new leadership approaches need to be implemented to effectively manage this new structure [46]. Developments in the field of management-organization and organizational behavior and new concepts have also led to the emergence of new leadership styles in leadership [4]. Leadership is important for every organization as well as for health organizations, because the success of an organization is a good leader [47]. For effective leadership, it is important to focus on the dynamic relationships between guidance, leadership values, culture, talent, and organizational context [48]. Effective leaders in health care services consider safe, qualified, and friendly care as the top priority. Effective leadership is critical to facilitate quality care, patient safety, and positive staff development. Leaders make the voice of patients continuous; they continuously monitor their patient experiences, concerns, needs, and feedback [49]. Nurses, the largest workforce in a health institution and a dynamic profession, play an important role in health leadership and policy-making, while maintaining their traditional care skills [50]. The leadership style of executive nurses plays an important role in the provision of job satisfaction and motivation of nurses, development of institutional commitment, and effective management of conflicts [51–53]. In addition, effective leadership styles can increase the quality of health care outcomes. In addition, leadership in health facilities is considered as an important factor in ensuring quality health services, patient satisfaction, and financial performance.

4. Conclusion

Nurses are responsible for guiding the community because of their responsibilities in health care. Patient care and education, effective communication, and clinical management are the most important tasks. These tasks are closely related to leadership behavior. Nurses who exhibit leadership behavior will be pioneers in bringing the profession to a professional level. The goal of future health care institutions should be to influence the quality of patient care through a good nursing leadership. Future research should focus on the development, applicability, and implementation of robust leadership style models in different health environments. These studies should include multidisciplinary professional teams; strengthen the role of nurses and other health professionals; and address organizational parameters and individual wishes, preferences, and expectations for quality of life and health care.

Acknowledgements

We thank everyone who provided scientific guidance.

Conflict of interest

The authors declare no conflict of interest.

Author details

Serpil Çelik Durmuş[1*] and Kamile Kırca[2]

1 Nursing Management Department, Faculty of Health Sciences, Kırıkkale University, Kırıkkale, Turkey

2 Nursing Department, Faculty of Health Sciences, Kırıkkale University, Kırıkkale, Turkey

*Address all correspondence to: serpilcelik2010@gmail.com

References

[1] Darzi, A. High Quality Care For All: NHS Next Stage Review Final Report. [Internet]. 2008. Available from: https://www.gov.uk/government/publications/high-quality-care-for-all-nhs-next-stage-review-final-report

[2] Keklik B. Determination of leadership types adopted in health services: A special hospital case. Afyon Kocatepe university. FEAS Journal. 2012;**14**(1):73-93

[3] Sfantou DF, Laliotis A, Patelarou AE, Pistollo DS, Matalliotakis M, Patelarou E. Importance of leadership style towards quality of care measures in healthcare settings: A systematic review. Healthcare. 2017;**5**(73):2-17

[4] Eryeşil K, İraz RA. Field study on the relationship between leadership styles and organizational commitment. Journal of Selçuk University Vocational School of Social Sciences. 2017;**20**(2):129-139

[5] Karahan A. Investigation of the relationship between leadership and organizational commitment in hospitals. Journal of Social Sciences. 2008;**10**(1):145-162

[6] Uysal ŞA, Keklik B, Erdem R, Çelik R. Investigation of the relationships between hospital Managers' leadership traits and work productivity levels of employees. Hacettepe Journal of Health Administration. 2012;**15**(1):25-56

[7] Koçel T. Business Management: Management and Organization, Behavior in Organizations, Classical, Modern, Contemporary and Contemporaneus Approaches. 10th ed. Istanbul: Beta Edition Publishing; 2005

[8] Sabuncuoglu Z, Tüz M. Organizational Psychology. Alfa Actual Distribution: Bursa; 2008

[9] Asamani JA, Naab F, Ofei AMA. Leadership styles in nursing management: Implications for staff outcomes. Journal of Health Science. 2016;**6**(1):23-36. DOI: 10.17532/jhsci.2016.266

[10] Cummings G. Editorial: Your leadership style – How are you working to achieve a preferred future? Journal of Clinical Nursing. 2012;**21**(23-24):3325-3327

[11] Cope V, Murray M. Leadership styles in nursing. Nursing Standard. 2017;**31**(43):61-70. DOI: 10.7748/ns.2017.e10836

[12] Anonson J, Walker ME, Arries E, Maposa S, Telford P, Berry L. Qualities of exemplary nurse leaders: Perspectives of frontline nurses. Journal of Nursing Management. 2014;**22**(1):127-136

[13] Brewer C, Kovner C, Djukic M, Fatehi F, Greene W, Chacko TP, et al. Impact of transformational leadership on nurse work outcomes. Journal of Advanced Nursing. 2016;**72**(11):2879-2893

[14] Intestines AS, Peace VK. The effects of transformational and Interactionist leadership relationships on nursing and health services. ACU Health Information Journal. 2018;**9**(2):97-104

[15] Brendel W, Bennett C. Learning to embody leadership through mindfulness and somatics practice. Advances in Developing Human Resources. 2016;**18**(3):409-425

[16] Laschinger HK, Wong CA, Cummings GG, Grau AL. Resonant leadership and workplace empowerment: The value of positive organisational cultures in reducing workplace incivility. Nursing Economics. 2014;**32**(1):5-15

[17] World Health Organisation (WHO). Open Mındsets: Partıcıpatory Leadershıp For Health. WHO Library Cataloguing-in-Publication Data. Available from: http://www.who.int, France, 2016, 1-30

[18] Giltinane CL. Leadership styles and theories. Nursing Standard. 2013;**27**(41):35-39

[19] Dilek H. Leadership Styles and Perception of Justice; a Research on Effects of Organizational Commitment, Job Satisfaction and Organizational Citizenship Behavior. Gebze: Gebze Institute of Technology; 2005

[20] Marquis BL, Huston CJ. Leadership and Management Tools for the New Nurse: A Case Study Approach. Philadelphia PA: Lippincott Williams & Wilkins; 2012

[21] Akyurt N, Alpaslan M, Oktar ÖF. Leadership styles in health workers-job satisfaction-organizational commitment model. Süleyman Demirel University Visionary Journal. 2015;**6**(13):50-61

[22] Zhu W, Sosik JJ, Riggio RE, Yang B. Relationships between transformational and active transactional leadership and followers' organizational identification: The role of psychological empowerment. Journal of Behavioral and Applied Management. 2012;**13**(3):186-212

[23] Bass BM, Steidlmeier P. Ethics, character, and authentic transformational leadership behavior. The Leadership Quarterly. 1999;**10**(2):181-217

[24] Sosik JJ, Jung DD. Full Range Leadership Development: Pathways for People, Profit and Planet. New York: Taylor & Francis; 2011

[25] Kılıç R, Keklik B, Yildiz H. A study aimed at determining the effect of transformative and fully free leadership styles on organizational silence. Management and Economics. 2014;**21**(2):249-268

[26] Bish M. Leadership and management frameworks and theories. In: Day GE, Leggat SG, editors. Leading and Managing Health Services: An Australasian Perspective. Port Melbourne: Cambridge University Press; 2015. pp. 16-28

[27] Bach S, Ellis P. Leadership, Management and Team Working in Nursing Transforming Nursing Practice Series. Exeter, UK: Learning Matters; 2011

[28] Barlı Ö. Behavioral Sciences and Behavior in Organizations. 3rd ed. Istanbul: Aktif Publishing House; 2008

[29] Bass BM. Does the transactional–transformational leadership paradigm transcend organizational and National Boundaries? American Psychologist. 1997;**52**(2):130-139

[30] Northouse PG. Leadership, Theory and Practices. 6th ed. Istanbul: Surat Univercity Publishing, Trans. Cengiz Simsek; 2014

[31] Şentürk FK, Durak M, Yılmaz E, Kaban T, Kök N, Baş AA. Study on determining the effects of transformational and Interactionist leadership styles on individual innovation. Mehmet Akif Ersoy University Journal of Social Science Institute. 2016;**8**(17):173-198

[32] Bass BM, Avolio BJ, Jung DI, Berson Y. Predicting unit performance by assessing transformational and transactional leadership. Journal of Applied Psychology. 2003;**88**(2):207-218. DOI: 10.1037/0021-9010.88.2.207

[33] Tengilimoglu D. A field study to determine the characteristics of leadership behavior in public

and private sector organizations. Electronic Journal of Social Sciences. 2005;**4**(14):1-16

[34] Tengilimoglu D, Yigit A. A field study on the effect of leadership behaviors on personnel job satisfaction in hospitals. Hacettepe Journal of Health Administration. 2005;**8**(3):374-400

[35] Schoel C, Bluemke M, Mueller P, Stahlberg D. When autocratic leaders become an option--uncertainty and self-esteem predict implicit leadership preferences. Journal of Personality and Social Psychology. 2011;**101**(3):521-540. DOI: 10.1037/a0023393

[36] Arun K. Leadership Styles and Sharing Knowledge Relationship. Erzurum: Ataturk University, Institute of Social Sciences; 2008

[37] Minister I, Büyükbese T. Leadership types and current-future situation comparison of power sources: A field research based on the perceptions of the administrators of educational institutions. Karamanoglu Mehmetbey University Journal of Social and Economic Research. 2010;**12**(19):73-84

[38] Telli E, Unsar SA, Oguzhan A. The effects of leadership behavioral styles on Employees' organizational burnout and displacement tendencies: A case study. Electronic Journal of Vocational Colleges. 2012;**2**(2):135-150

[39] Çetin T. The Effect of Fully Free Leadership Understanding on Innovation Trends of Mid-Term Managers: An Application in Furniture Enterprises in the Aegean Region. Unpublished Master Thesis, Dumlupınar University Institute of Social Sciences, Kütahya, 2009

[40] Skogstad A, Einarsen S, Torsheim T, Aasland MS, Hetland H. The destructiveness of laissez-faire leadership behavior. Journal of Occupational Health Psychology. 2007;**12**(1):80-92

[41] Hinkin TR, Schriesheim CA. An examination of nonleadership: From Laissezfaire leadership to leader reward omission and punishment omission. Journal of Applied Psychology. 2008;**93**(6):1234-1248

[42] Chaudhry AQ, Javed H. Impact of transactional and laissez faire leadership style on motivation. International Journal of Business and Social Science. 2012;**3**(7):258-264

[43] Antonakis J, House R. On İnstrumental Leadership: Beyond Transactions and Transformations. Omaha: UNL Gallup Leadership Institute Summit; 2004

[44] Hooijberg R, Antonakis J. Instrumental Leadership: The Nuts and Bolts of Leadership. [Internet]. 2014. Available from: www.imd.org/globalassets/publications/insightsimd/docs/38---instrumental-leadership.pdf [Accessed: 31-05-2017]

[45] Kılınç T. Developments in situational leadership: Developments in leadership approach. Istanbul University Journal of Faculty of Business Administration. 1995;**24**(1):59-76

[46] Dodson D. What's the Best Leadership Style for Healthcare? Leadership and Workforce Development. [İnternet]. 2017. Available from: https://nchica.org/whats-the-best-leadership-style-for-healthcare

[47] Ballow C. Leaders and Systems. The Governance Institute White Paper. Winter 2009. 1-2

[48] Al-Sawai A. Leadership of healthcare professionals: Where do we stand? Oman Medical Journal. 2013;**28**(4).285-287

[49] Gün İ, Aslan Ö. Leadership theories and leadership in health business. Journal of Health and Nursing Management. 2018;**5**(3):217-226

[50] Cherian S, Karkada S. Review on leadership in nursing. International Journal of Nursing Research and Practice. 2017;**4**(1):57-66

[51] Kurt SD. The Effect of Leadership Behaviors of Clinical Responsible Nurses on Nurses' Job Satisfaction. (Thesis). Halic University, Institute of Health Sciences. İstanbul. 2009

[52] Bucak B. The Perceptions of Leadership Approaches and Conflict Management Strategies of Nurses Who Work in Two Different Hospitals in Ankara. (Thesis). Gazi University Institute of Health Sciences. Ankara. 2010

[53] Gülkaya G. Transformative Leadership Behaviors of Nurses in Service and Motivation Status of Nurses Working Together. (Thesis). Hacettepe University, Institute of Health Sciences. Ankara. 2012

Chapter 2

Simulation: A Training Resource for Quality Care and Improving Patient Safety

Eliana Escudero, Marlova Silva and Marcia Corvetto

Abstract

Patient safety is an ever-present topic in the discussion of educators. It has been 20 years since the publication of *To Err Is Human*, and there are lessons learned, although there is still much to be done. Healthcare systems are becoming increasingly complex, putting the safety of patients at risk. In this context, there is a greater exposure of healthcare professionals to medical-legal liability issues and to becoming victims of situations that are often preventable. Nurses and medical doctors are especially exposed to these situations, since they are visible during procedures, or do so during the points of greater risk during the patient care process. This chapter will review the contribution provided by the curricular integration of simulation-based education as a tool to train technical and nontechnical issues and how this work can be done for the safety of patients through a standardized training plan, under controlled and evaluated processes. We will discuss how resources and elements allow to perform healthcare interventions in a more safely manner. Finally, we will review the existing literature, some experiences, and the available evidence on this topic.

Keywords: patient safety, collaboration, communication, innovation, quality of care

1. Introduction

Nowadays patient safety is a very important topic in healthcare. Healthcare systems are becoming increasingly complex, putting at risk the safety of our patients. In this context, there is a greater exposure of healthcare professionals to medical-legal liability issues. Secondary to this situation, healthcare educators have incorporated this topic into the curriculum of healthcare careers.

As in other areas of human endeavor, such as commercial and military aviation, simulation has provided an opportunity to prepare teams. Teams have the opportunity to practice skills and work through complex situations before facing the real environment, aiming to achieve safety and to prevent the incidence of errors. Mistakes in healthcare can harm patients and also affect professionals and institutions, which can be frustrated, questioned, and sanctioned.

Crisis situations and the complexity of work systems in healthcare can be recreated in simulated environments with the same level of realism as it may occur in real clinical setting. The benefit is that the activity happens in a protected environment, allowing the occurrence of mistakes, their analysis, and reflection. These scenarios also review group behavior and the implementation of protocols up to the point where there is certainty in the fact that teams could make decisions and are prepared to face real-world conditions. In a simulated environment, error becomes an opportunity to learn and to achieve competencies, which will imply a reduction of incidents and adverse outcomes.

This chapter will provide information about the methodology of simulation-based education, about international standards in clinical simulation and will develop concepts of human factor and patient safety. It shall review the new role of educators and the challenges during healthcare professional training, focusing on physicians and nurses, since they are the most exposed during patient care. Finally, we will also present some methods and assessment tools to evaluate and analyze the current impact of simulation.

The purpose of this chapter is to provide evidence using simulation and experiences identifying how to improve professional competencies, in a time when it is necessary to incorporate new methodologies of education and technologies and innovate toward efficiency and effectiveness, making the process safer toward a culture of safety.

In summary, the authors want to contribute to the knowledge in the field of clinical simulation, patient safety, and safe nursing care, because today is mandatory for clinical teams and healthcare students to have these competencies.

2. Education-based simulation and definitions

Significant changes in clinical attention are being observed worldwide. This evolution has not been without issues, but also has been surrounded by opportunities for innovation. The increased pace of research, growing of knowledge, and progress in technology have contributed to improve the life expectancy of people. Additionally, there are new challenges, such as incoming chronic and infectious diseases, environmental hazards, and demographic and epidemiological transitions. In this scenario, the main challenge for nurses and healthcare professionals is to contribute to deliver safer attention in this increasingly complex and unsafe patient's environment.

On the other hand, those committed to undergraduate, postgraduate, and continuing medical education and train of healthcare professionals must deliver answers to this complex scenario, with fast and continuous changes in the paradigm of teaching and learning [1]. There is a lack of coordination between the competencies that graduates achieve during their careers and the real needs of the clinical environment of healthcare. Graduates need to train technical skills, have more time for clinical practice, and have more chances to interact with real patients. High-quality and efficient healthcare attention requires professionals capable to work immersed in interprofessional teams, with a high degree of leadership and decision-making skills [1].

In this context, the role of nursing is essential. It is a profession that promotes patient safety and, at the same time, guarantees high-quality medical attention. In places where education education and training of these professionals is fundamental to generate changes in the safety culture of institutions [2].

The intervention of healthcare education through the integration of active and innovative methodologies and the strengthening of the relationship between academia and healthcare area are some strategies that have been developed in order to solve this issue.

Many interventions have been described in order to develop these competencies: the use of technologies, virtual tools, problem-based learning, interprofessional education, and specially clinical simulation [3].

In order to clear the concepts of patient safety and simulation-based education, it is important to state some definitions.

Some relevant definitions of simulation are:

- As per Lopreiato: "A strategy in which a particular set of conditions are created or replicated to resemble authentic situations that are possible in real life. Simulation can incorporate one or more modalities to promote, improve, or validate a participant's performance" [4].

- "Created or replicated to resemble authentic situations that are possible in real life. Simulation can incorporate one or more modalities to promote, improve, or validate a participant's performance" [5].

- "Clinical simulation is a technique, not a technology, that substitutes or broadens a real experience through a guided experience that emulates or replicates aspects of the real world in an interactive manner" [6].

- "Methodology that creates a situation or environment in order to allow the people participating in it to experience a realistic representation of a healthcare situation with the purpose of practice, learning, evaluate or work over aspects of communication and leadership" [7].

A simple definition of Patient Safety by the WHO is "Prevention of errors and adverse effects to patients associated with health care" [8].

Primum non nocere (first, to do no harm) is a basic concept in healthcare. Numerous worldwide studies conducted since the year 2000 show how patients may be harmed as a result of healthcare attention with an important percentage of preventability [9]. A *learning curve* makes reference to a period of time an individual takes to learn a subject or specific skill. This learning period can increase the potential percentage of events resulting in harm for real patients; therefore, it is a priority to implement learning models that do not expose patients to this risk. There is compelling evidence regarding how educational interventions with clinical simulation allow healthcare professionals to acquire knowledge, skills, and behaviors, having a positive impact on patient safety [10]. A paper written by Mary Ann Cantrell allows us to become familiar with studies that show how simulation methodology has an impact on cognitive and procedural outcomes, not only in undergraduate nursing students but also in professionals [11].

Many different classifications of simulation devices exist [12, 13]. The spectrum of clinical simulators includes part-task trainers, computer-based systems, virtual reality and haptic systems, simulated patients, simulated environments, and integrated simulators (both, model- and instructor-driven simulators). The choice of the simulator will depend on the competition or the skill the instructor wants to train [12].

Regarding fidelity of simulation, many different definitions exist too [14]. Following the definitions of the Sim-dictionary developed by the SSH [4], low-fidelity simulation is not needing to be controlled or programmed externally for the learner to participate; examples include case studies, role playing, or task trainers used to support students or professionals in learning a clinical situation or practice. That type of simulation activities called low fidelity requires the educator's feedback. Some examples are intravenous catheter insertion, drug administration, or introduction of a urine catheter.

The other one is high fidelity and refers to simulation experiences that are extremely realistic and provide a high level of interactivity and realism for the learner. This definition can apply to any mode or method of simulation; for example: human, manikin, task trainer, or virtual reality.

High fidelity uses full-body manikins with computers that give very realistic physiology answers to train nontechnical skills. This modality allows to train leadership and make safe decisions, teamwork, and communication. An example is training for advance CPR. High fidelity simulation ended with a reflexion named "Debriefing", that is the most important part of simulation. Debriefing is for collecting information, a reflection in team about the experience to improve for the next time.

With these types and levels of simulation, this methodology allows both, individual and team training, showing an improvement in the performance of healthcare systems, lowering the incidence of errors and improving the quality of healthcare [15].

There are three domains where clinical simulation may be used by healthcare professionals [10]:

1. Practice and evaluation of technical skills through various models or software developed for that purpose.

2. Practice with a simulated patient to develop communicational skills.

3. Training of teams who face critical situations through the implementation of high-fidelity scenarios, which are characterized by having an extremely high degree of realism, allowing for high interactivity among the participating individuals. This type of scenario is followed by an after-action review, better known as debriefing [4].

3. Values and beginning of simulation-based education

This section presents the main historical events associated with clinical simulation and its value, based on models and theoretical framework that support it. We will review international standards for their implementation, essential elements that have made it a powerful tool regarding patient safety:

3.1 Clinical simulation as a teaching and learning methodology

Since over four decades, the use of clinical simulation as a valuable methodology has shown an important growth worldwide. Its implementation in nursing and other healthcare professions was adopted from other industries known as High Reliability Organizations, which are characterized by operating in complex high-risk contexts, showing low rates of accidents, failures, or catastrophic events. These organizations, such as aviation, electricity, and nuclear energy, are based on five fundamental pillars, being one of them the training of personnel through the use of simulation methodology [16].

Sim One, *Harvey*, and *Resusci Anne* were the first simulators which over five decades ago were designed with interactive characteristics to enable the development of certain skills in the training of healthcare professionals. Currently there are a large variety of resources that have allowed for clinical simulation to become a gold standard and a valuable and essential methodology for the process of teaching and learning in healthcare careers.

Simulation has been developed around the world, with various degrees of development, involving scientific societies in the fields of academia, research, and program accreditation. Simulations allow an important collaborative and networking job between countries and organizations [17].

The value of simulation as a methodology is provided in no small measure by the models and theoretical frameworks that support it; the most relevant are described below:

Andragogy: It refers to the learning theory of how adults learn. Professionals who work in the field of healthcare are adults that base their learning in the main principles of andragogy: internal motivation, a taste for problem-solving, autonomy, exacting standards, preference for practical activities, and previous experience. Clinical simulation as a methodology enables learning by respecting each one of these principles, which enhances its value in the training of professionals for the improvement of patient safety [18].

Deliberate practice: This theory on an experience that allows for the accomplishment of a competence through systematic and controlled practice, allowing the learner to have a full awareness of their progress and achievements. When deliberate practice is carried out through clinical simulation, it allows to learn by means of repetition, without sacrificing patient safety. This theory is also known as the expert theory, which states that expertise goes beyond a genetic condition, being a person, through practice, able to achieve its maximum potential in a given field [3].

David Kolb: This theory states that through concrete and active experience, based on reflection, the individual who performs a training activity with simulation can achieve behavioral changes through abstract conceptualization [3].

Dreyfus and Dreyfus: This theory states that every professional in the field of nursing or other healthcare profession goes through five stages that range from novice to expert professional. Simulation as a methodology strengthens the transition through these stages from undergraduate training to continuing education in highly experienced professionals [19].

Reflective practice (Schön): This theory formulates that reflection is essential for learning. All learning practices must include a moment of reflection that accompanies the performed action. Feedback and debriefing are the intentional reflexive methods that accompany a clinical simulation experience, during and after the action where the educator can verify learning achievements [20].

3.2 International standards for the implementation of teaching based on clinical simulation

In the academic environment, the need to implement and evaluate the integration of simulation methodology in the educational processes arises. The training of these new educators with quality tools and evidence-based standards is also necessary.

The development and implementation of standards allows for continuous improvement based on established benchmarks, and it is through the work of experts and scientific societies around the world, such as the National League for Nursing (NLN), the International Nursing Association for Clinical Simulation and Learning [21], and the Society for Simulation in Healthcare (SSH), among others. These are the bases to begin with tools which establish and give the reference frameworks, glossaries, codes of ethics, good practice standards, and research topics. They created this methodology, allowing subsequent growth and development.

Below are the main implementation standards recommended for teaching based on clinical simulation:

3.3 National League for Nursing accreditation standards

Dedicated to excellence in nursing, the National League for Nursing is the premier organization for nurse faculty and leaders in nursing education [22]. The NLN offers professional development, networking opportunities, testing services, nursing research grants, and public policy. NLN members represent nursing education programs across the spectrum of higher education, healthcare organizations, and agencies.

The NLN promotes global excellence standards in the field of nursing education through a process of accreditation that respects the diversity of the mission statement of a program, study plans, learners, and faculty, with the objective of implementing a culture of continuous improvement in the field of nursing education.

Its standards are:

- Standard I: Culture of Excellence—Program Outcomes
- Standard II: Culture of Integrity and Accountability—Mission, Governance, and Resources
- Standard III: Culture of Excellence and Caring—Faculty
- Standard IV: Culture of Excellence and Caring—Students
- Standard V: Culture of Learning and Diversity—Curriculum and Evaluation Processes

3.4 SSH accreditation standards

The purpose of the Society for Simulation in Healthcare is to serve a global community of practice enhancing the quality of healthcare [23]. This society has an international accreditation program that considers five areas of accreditation, each one with defined criteria:

- Core
- Assessment
- Research
- Teaching/education
- System integration

3.5 International Nursing Association for Clinical Simulation and Learning Standards (INACSL)

The mission of this society is "To advance the science of healthcare simulation" [24].

The latest official standards of this organization include recommendations for:

- Simulation design
- Outcomes and objectives

- Facilitation
- Debriefing
- Participant evaluation
- Professional integrity
- Simulation-enhanced IPE
- Operations

4. Patient safety concepts and curriculum integration in health careers

Patient safety has been recognized as a fundamental right, which has been expressed in various laws and declarations, and we must strive toward it [25, 26].

Patient safety was branded as a universal concept in 2004 [25]. The English physician Dr Liam Donaldson, based on the book *To Err is Human*, decides to create the World Alliance for Patient Safety under the wing of the World Health Organization [25]. This group proposes, as its first objective, to coordinate, disseminate, and accelerate around the world all improvements related to patient safety, sharing common strategies and standardized procedures around the world. This work produces the "Hand Hygiene" protocol (Indications for Hand Hygiene) [27], known and applied around the world. Another major contribution was the creation of the protocol for surgical safety pause [28]. Likewise, many other subjects have been developed by the World Alliance, whose objective is to achieve patient safety and low cost and high satisfaction on the achieved objectives.

One of the relevant results emerging from this work is to have a unique definition for patient safety, which allows us to enable a series of actions and interventions around the world that stem from this concept. We shall now review the latest definition, which was worked on and discussed at length, over several months, by the community of the WHO Patient Safety Network, and published in 2018.

"Patient safety is the absence of preventable harm to a patient during the process of health care and reduction of risk of unnecessary harm associated with health care to an acceptable minimum. An acceptable minimum refers to the collective notions of given current knowledge, resources available and the context in which care was delivered weighed against the risk of non-treatment or other treatment" [25]. This definition is quite similar to the previous one; however, resources and context become relevant, including the concepts of knowledge and update. We can therefore consider as a self-evident truth that, in the face of development and the availability of technological and academic conditions for education, the use of simulation-based training is a valuable and increasingly affordable alternative.

Dr Liam Donaldson remains to this day a leader in this subject and has developed a global work agenda that already has experts among its ranks that through virtual networks communicate and organize subgroups and commissions in permanent development of initiatives. There are events and congresses, societies with strategic projects, and preset goals to be fulfilled within defined timelines. They are looking for common results that, if achieved, shall be highly impactful with a global scope. Within the World Alliance objectives declared for 2016–2025 period, we find reducing medication errors that now comprise one of the leading causes of death [29] and also damage caused. This problem has not been sufficiently researched, but we can infer that harm and damages are also high, many of which could be preventable if the strategy is strong and known for all. This is a concern for many different countries and groups around the world. All the above also implies elevated costs to society, which may be better used in research, new hospitals, and vaccines, every one of them very worthy of consideration in the field of healthcare. However, work on patient safety is not only an exclusive concern of the clinical field but is also arising in the context of academia, where it is fundamental to prepare students from healthcare careers, making them safe professionals. This is increasingly more demanding on account of the legal aspects of healthcare, and a more active participation of patients and their families in sanitary issues, and their role when facing medical decisions. In the book *To Err Is Human*, the need to incorporate the use of clinical simulation is first established [30]. It presents a proposal that shall lead directly to a change in paradigm in education, since it shall be acceptable that errors occur, and to avoid or diminish their impact, they must be analyzed. We can point out and recognize that this is a starting and inflection point toward change and therefore also the moment for integrating the methodology into the environment of healthcare. At that time this was an innovative idea, which was not being applied in human health area. Nevertheless, during the decade of the 1960s, we can already find evidence of a small successful result by means of simulation. As it was previously stated, this wasn't either the first proposal for its use in a clinical setting; however, due to various reasons, it had not prospered, and only from the year 2000 clinical simulation is associated with the subject of error, which is still a very complex topic. From this moment onward, various initiatives are generated around the world, from where leaders emerge, mobilizing clinicians and educators to this day. Worth mentioning are David Gaba, anesthesiologist and a pioneer of simulation techniques for crisis management in Stanford, known as the Crisis Resource Management [31]; Dr Peter Dieckmann, who from the area of psychology has researched and analyzed debriefing models; and lastly Dr Pamela Jeffries, nurse and a renowned leader on account of her theoretical model and her contributions to society through her research in the area of clinical simulation.

Also, along the same lines, scientific societies emerge, which now call professionals from around the world to attend events and dedicate their work to the training of simulation methods and evidence gathering, such as SSH and INACSL, among others previously described.

It has been nearly 20 years devoted to becoming aware of the need for change. The World Health Organization, in 2010, proposed a curriculum for the training of midwives and nurses, highlighting the need for simulation laboratories at the same level of classrooms and libraries [32].

Around the same time, in 2009, the curricular safety guidelines for medical students and in 2011 for other professionals are made available [25], which again propose the integration of simulation in training.

These documents are the fruit of the work and data collection by experts, which makes clear the need to intervene and generate change.

The nursing profession has led the way around the world, garnering momentum for a movement in favor of the advancement in the integration of simulation in curricular proposals.

This is how educational projects, which have been successful around the world, on different continents, mainly the United States, Australia, and the Nordic countries, are initiated. It should be noted that the integration of simulation in study programs requires work oriented to obtaining measurable and observable results that allow proposing continuous improvement, in which the role of the teacher is key to the success of the experience [33]. Carrying out planned work, along with the development of a series of tools to be considered as guides, rubrics, and guidelines, as well as a permanent training plan, an institutional strategic plan, and a continuous reflective look, makes this methodology a permanent challenge. Considering that the authors are from Chile and they have developed their experience in countries of the region, it is possible to point out that there are already successful integration experiences in undergraduate programs in nursing and some, but in smaller numbers, in medicine; in graduate and postgraduate degrees, they are still very scarce. It is therefore an interesting moment to carry out research and generate reports of the results achieved to date.

5. Patient safety and relationship with human factors

The book *To Err Is Human* raises the issue of the complexity of the work system in the environment of healthcare, which is generated by various reasons, such as the multiplicity of simultaneous events, interruptions, fatigue, work flows, etc., and illustrates this in a model that is used today to explain the phenomenon that is known as the *theory of Reason* (after James T. Reason, of the University of Manchester) or of the *Swiss cheese model*. The remarkable thing about this way of presenting the processes in a system, in this case from a sanitary standpoint, is how didactical it is to better understand errors. The image of the Swiss cheese allows observing that between processes multiple instances arise in which there are possible breaks of safety controls. The field of engineering has always worked considering that error is part of their work, and, as pointed out by Mavilde da Luz Gonçalves Pedreira in her book *Nursing on a Daily Basis: Patient Safety* published in 2011, the engineer trains for this eventuality and creates intervention and safety points in risk areas, constantly evaluating and measuring, with optimal results for the user. However, this does not occur in healthcare where, for example, we do not have rigorous induction and orientation processes in place, which in other industries are known as "trainee programs." Our working day is normally long and many times needs to be extended beyond human capacity. The feedback loops are not in place; there is no testing of protocols; there is a lack of both guidelines for checking any of the above and reflection times for decision-making, which in our region are also part of a very hierarchical and compartmentalized cultural issue. All of this is known as the human factor, meaning the integration between the organization, work itself, and staff, which has been studied deeply by sociologists and ergonomists [34]. It is still today a subject that is rarely discussed by administrative staff and the managers of clinical institutions and integrated into the programs and curriculum of healthcare careers in most countries of the world. However, today is part of the terminology of the Sim-dictionary, and this has two major foundations [4]. The first is what the WHO points out in 2004 in its publication *Learning by Errors* in which it is emphatic to declare that this is a subject that should always be taught but that we see that it is mostly unknown [35]. And the second is provided by the objective of simulation, whose purpose is to work for the safety of the patient, and it is Dr. Gaba, recognized for his work in crisis management and expertise in high-fidelity scenarios, who states that in the performance of professionals, they are exposed to certain critical points [36], which are all associated with the elements present in the human factor concept; therefore they are not only technical issues but also of systematic, in which, for various reasons, human behavior can put safety at risk. One of his last publications, *Human Factors Engineering in Patient Safety* [37], allows to finally unite the world of engineering with healthcare and raises an interesting proposal of the intervention of engineers and the resources of their discipline for simulations, in a capacity of trained experts who can suggest how to avoid breakpoints in the safety chain through simulations designed by a multidisciplinary team.

As previously stated, it is Dr Gaba, an anesthesiologist from Stanford University, United States, who incorporates into simulation a tool already used in the field of aviation, which first he adapts to anesthesia and subsequently implements for general clinical activity, called Crisis Resource Management or CRM [38]. This modality, which is carried out in very realistic scenarios, identifies 15 key points that, according to what Gaba observed in his institution, generate the most errors [39]. It should be noted that one of them, effective communication, is the key issue that has been analyzed, investigated, and evidenced by many, being considered as the one that triggers the most errors. This implies, therefore, that it is essential to train as teams in simple and complex scenarios where the element of crisis allows to look for individual and collective safe behaviors, which after being analyzed through debriefing will allow to achieve good performance objectives in a shared, and therefore safe, manner.

6. Learning activities to teach safety competencies with simulation

To conduct the curricular integration of the methodology is not currently an easy subject for academics and clinicians. It implies changes of the teaching paradigm, mainly by a new role of the teacher that in addition to be a healthcare professional must be familiar with medical education or education in health sciences. The simulation educator or simulationist, which requires at least 2 years of training, must carry out his/her work under standards of simulation education applying new teaching tools such as feedback, coaching, reflection, deliberate practice, and others [24]. The simulationist must guide their teaching toward the learning outcomes and not only from the designed objective, understanding that this methodology should be used in all required levels, that is, undergraduate, postgraduate, and continuing education [4, 40].

There are models designed to implement this proposal; however, the most complex aspect of this is that this frame of reference is designed from the curriculum project of the unit, which implies serious and profound interventions [41]. Without this, it is not feasible that the process responds to the profiles of graduates, postgraduate, or specialty programs. Let us remember that any curricular intervention requires logic and a coordination of all the educational strategies to be developed, making it unique and respond to a construction not only of contents or disciplinary elements.

We present below the models of two of the authors of this chapter, which have been constructed based on the units responsible for the integration projects of the simulation. It is interesting, given that the first is the result of a curricular project designed for the school of nursing of the Finis Terrae University of Chile (**Figure 1**) and the second from San Sebastian University of Chile (**Figure 2**). Even though they have two different origins, they share a series of elements that are transversal to any current simulation proposal.

It seems important to point out and recommend to clinicians other instances of the application of the simulation, such as simulation in situ. This application of simulation is understood as one performed in the real setting, that is, in the clinical environment with its physical resources, equipment, and systems, in addition to its protocols, routines, and usual work teams to be trained [42]. The purpose of this modality of simulation is mainly oriented to safety, and one of its proposals is aimed at training teams to identify latent safety threats in their work environments. Simulation in situ is a newer modality than simulation in centers and must solve issues such as spaces, times, fears from professionals, and contamination of

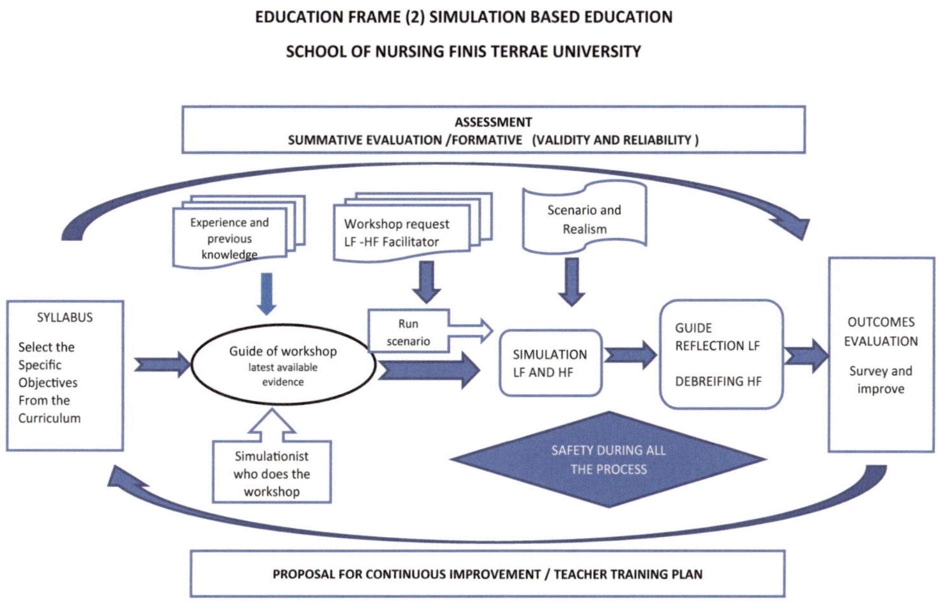

Figure 1.
Frame of simulation from nursing of the Finis Terrae University of Chile.

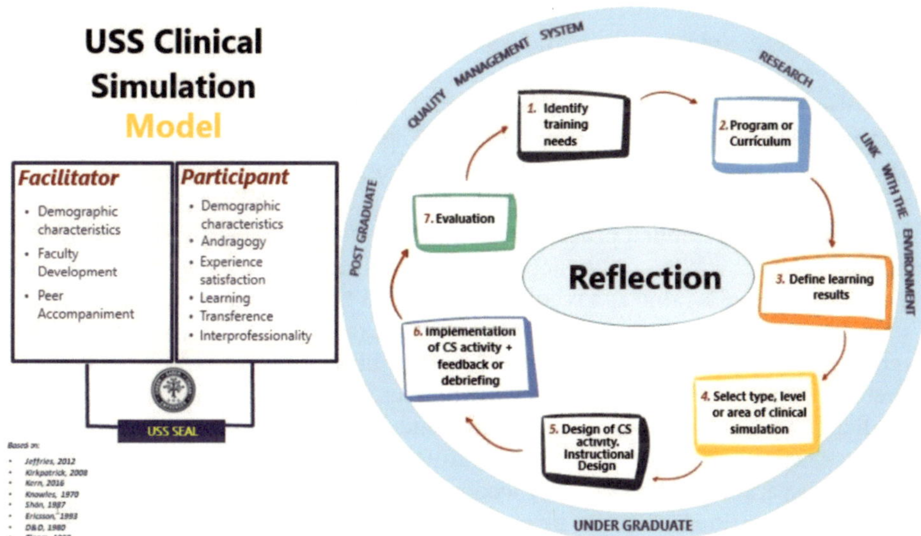

Figure 2.
Frame of simulation from San Sebastian University of Chile.

simulators, among others. The experiences carried out have been well evaluated, for example, in the cases of hospital emergencies, although there is still much to be developed and researched in this regard [43].

6.1 Strategies and tools

Many systematic approaches have been developed in order to achieve an effective teamwork and communication in healthcare. One example of these strategies for patient safety is SBAR: Situation-Background-Assessment-Recommendation. This is a tool that provides a framework for communication between members of the healthcare team about a patient's condition. This instrument is useful in emergency or for giving information through a phone call, for example. It has been used successfully in clinical environment [44]. The school of nursing from Finis Terrae uses and trains the students with SBAR. The students are prepared to phone the physicians or a colleague and summarize all the most important information about the case and the patient. The students do for several times during the career to be ready and sure.

Another resource that is necessary to mention is Team Strategies and Tools to Enhance Performance and Patient Safety (TeamSTEPPS). This strategy has been considered like a good model for training the teams, and part of this is doing with simulation and optimizing team performance across the healthcare delivery system [45].

7. How to assess competencies of safety patient with clinical simulation

According to the pyramid model described by Miller, we can assess learners at four different levels [46]. These levels are (1) knows (knowledge), (2) knows how (applied knowledge), (3) shows how (performance), and (4) does (action or behavior in real practice) [46]. Different methodologies have been used to evaluate these four different levels of competence. For example, if we want to assess trainees to "show how," the ACGME Toolbox of Assessment Methods suggests that simulations are the most appropriate methodology. One of the strengths of simulation as an assessment methodology is the high degree of reliability. We can present a situation in the same manner for every student, situation that becomes especially important for certification and recertification processes [47].

Regarding how to measure competence during simulations, many assessment tools have been described in the literature. Based on the literature related to simulation-based assessment, two types of observational scales have been described, explicit process and implicit process [48]. Explicit process scores take the form of commonly used checklists or key actions. Implicit process scoring is a tool where the entire performance is rated as a whole and is named global rating scales. In general, the choice of metrics will depend on what we want to measure. If we want to assess "technical" skills (airway management, drug administration, and placement of catheters), it is usually possible to identify key actions and to develop checklists. On the other hand, if we want to assess "nontechnical" skills such as communication, teamwork, and situation awareness, it is better to use global rating scales.

Regarding assessment tools for procedural skills, recent investigations suggest that global rating scales may be more sensitive in determining competence for procedural skills [49]. Ma and colleagues provide an example whereby the use of a global rating scale may be preferred over the use of two currently available checklists during central venous catheter placement [50]. Additionally, checklists have been unable to find differences between novices and experts [51]. A possible explanation is that knowledge acquisition through lectures, videos, or other material reviewed prior to the assessment session allowed novices to complete easily the majority of the key actions requested by the checklist from a cognitive standpoint. This interpretation challenges the utility of checklists as an assessment tool for procedural competences.

Additionally, more sensitive technical performance measurements, such as limb kinematics (trajectory, velocity, and acceleration), may provide additional performance assessment [52]. The use of these motion devices in the evaluation of motor skills allows obtaining quantitative data complementing previous validated visual scales [53]. Recent evidence supports their use in specific procedures. Clinkard provided evidence of construct validity for hand-motion-tracking analysis during US-guided CVC installation in a simulated setting. They concluded that motion analysis is a feasible tool for assessing competence in US-guided CVC, discriminating between performance level of novices and experts [54].

Regarding assessment tools for nontechnical skills (NTS), such as teamwork, communication, and decision-making, multiple tools have been developed over the last decades. A recent systematic review with the aim to analyze the context of use, method of development, evidence of validity, reliability, and usability of tools for the observer-based assessment of NTS in healthcare found 76 tools for assessment of NTS in healthcare [55]. The authors suggested a need for rationalization and standardization of the way we assess NTS in healthcare and greater consistency in how tools are developed and deployed.

In another systematic review aimed to synthesize available tools assessing teamwork performance of teams in crisis situations, 13 tools are identified for assessing teamwork of teams in crisis situations [56]. The tool TEAM may be the most promising tool given its measurement evidence [57]. Finally, they mentioned that there is a lack of tools to assess teamwork performance during intraoperative crisis situations [56].

8. Evidence regarding how simulation improves patient safety

Evaluating the patient impact of simulation-based education has become a priority in the present time. A recent review about using clinical simulation to study how to improve quality and safety in healthcare determined that using simulation in the study of healthcare improvement is a promising approach that could usefully complement established research method [58].

Simulation training in anesthesia has been used successfully and has shown to increase many skills of anesthesiologists. Nevertheless, there has not been a demonstrable improvement in patient outcomes with simulation training [59].

Unfortunately, systematic reviews indicate that patient outcomes are reported in only 0–5% of medical education studies [60]. Most of the simulation research body has focused on the performance of students, both in simulated environment and its transfer in the real patient. However, the impact of such simulated training, on the real patient outcomes, has been poorly studied.

A review on the evidence regarding educational interventions to enhance patient safety using a nontechnical skills training approach was published in 2012. A total of 22 studies met the inclusion criteria. There was a variation in the focus of outcomes among the studies, with representation of all levels of Kirkpatrick's adapted hierarchy. Only three measured patient outcomes. The methodological quality of published studies is reasonable, although the reporting of specific interventions is poor. There is a significant variation in the outcome measures used in this research, which limits the strength of conclusions on the effectiveness of these interventions [61].

A systematic review published by Zendejas identified 50 studies reporting patient outcomes in the evaluation of simulation-based education for health professionals [62]. All the studies included in this systematic review involved procedural skills training (airway management, gastrointestinal endoscopy, central venous catheter insertion). Most outcomes of this group of studies are procedural success rate and complications. Unfortunately, the minority of studies reported other patient outcomes such as survival and duration of hospitalization. Finally, a meta-analytic synthesis demonstrated small to moderate effects favoring simulation in comparison with no intervention and small nonsignificant effects favoring simulation in comparison with non-simulation instruction. The authors stated that simulation-based education is associated with downstream benefits on patient care.

9. Conclusion

Clinical simulation is a very valuable methodology for training, aimed at increasing patient safety. It is not a methodology that is proposed only for professional nurses, which motivated this chapter to be developed by a doctor and nurses.

Today simulation is considered an important option to achieve a safety culture, and evidence points out that it is a great contribution and it is very accepted by the new generations of health professionals. We must not forget that there are many groups working around the world to achieve this objective and also many initiatives that must be linked and associated through collaborative networks. A challenge that remains is to involve patients and let them know more about the subject and join in to be an active participant for their safety.

Author details

Eliana Escudero[1*], Marlova Silva[2] and Marcia Corvetto[3]

1 Diego Portales University, Santiago, Chile

2 San Sebastian University, Santiago, Chile

3 Pontificia Universidad Católica de Chile, Santiago, Chile

*Address all correspondence to: eliana.escudero@udp.cl

References

[1] Frenk J, Chen L, Bhutta ZA, Cohen J, Crisp N, Evans T, et al. Profesionales de la salud para el nuevo siglo: transformando la educación para fortalecer los sistemas de salud en un mundo interdependiente. Educación Médica. 2015;**16**(1):9-16. DOI: 10.1016/j.edumed.2015.04.011

[2] Rebollo Gomez P, Manso Perea C. Seguridad del paciente y buenas practicas. 1st ed. Madrid: Fuden; 2018

[3] Motola I, Devine LA, Chung HS, Sullivan JE, Issenberg SB. Simulation in healthcare education: A best evidence practical guide. AMEE Guide No. 82. Medical Teacher. 2013;**35**(10):e1511-e1530. DOI: 10.3109/0142159X.2013.818632

[4] Lopreiato JO, Downing D, Gammon W, Lioce L, Sittner B, Slot V, et al. Healthcare Simulation Dictionary. 2016; Retrieved from: http://www.ssih.org/dictionary

[5] Training Committee. American Society for Gastrointestinal Endoscopy. Training guideline for use of propofol in gastrointestinal endoscopy. Gastrointestinal Endoscopy. 2004;**60**(2):167-172. DOI: 10.1016/s0016-5107(04)01699-2

[6] Gaba DM. The future vision of simulation in health care. Quality & Safety in Health Care. 2004;**13**(Suppl 1):i2-i10. DOI: 10.1136/qhc.13.suppl_1.i2

[7] Alinier G. Developing high-Fidelity health care simulation scenarios: A guide for educators and professionals. Simulation and Gaming. 2010;**42**(1):9-26. DOI: 10.1177/1046878109355683

[8] Patient Safety by the WHO [Internet]. 2019. Available from: http://www.euro.who.int/en/health-topics/Health-systems/patient-safety

[9] Aranaz-Andrés JM, Aibar-Remón C, Limón-Ramírez R, Amarilla A, Restrepo FR, Urroz O, et al. Diseño del estudio IBEAS: prevalencia de efectos adversos en hospitales de Latinoamérica. Revista de Calidad Asistencial. 2011;**26**(3):194-200. DOI: 10.1016/j.cali.2010.12.001

[10] Aggarwal R, Mytton O, Derbrew M, Hananel D, Heydenburg M, Issenberg B, et al. Training and simulation for patient safety. Quality & Safety in Health Care. 2010;**19**(Suppl. 2):i34-i43. DOI: 10.1136/qshc.2009.038562

[11] Cantrell M, Franklin A, Leighton K, Carlson A. The evidence in simulation-based learning experiences in nursing education and practice: An umbrella review. Clinical Simulation in Nursing. 2017;**13**(12):634-667. DOI: 10.1016/j.ecns.2017.08.004

[12] Maran NJ, Glavin RJ. Low- to high-fidelity simulation - a continuum of medical education? Medical Education. 2003;**37**(Suppl. 1):22-28

[13] Kneebone R. Simulation in surgical training: Educational issues and practical implications. Medical Education. 2003;**37**(3):267-277

[14] Gaba DM. The future vision of simulation in healthcare. Simulation in Healthcare. 2007;**2**(2):126-135. DOI: 10.1097/01.SIH.0000258411.38212.32

[15] Vincent C, Moorthy K, Sarker SK, Chang A, Darzi AW. Systems approaches to surgical quality and safety: From concept to measurement. Annals of Surgery. 2004;**239**(4):475-482. DOI: 10.1097/01.sla.0000118753.22830.41

[16] Enya A, Dempsey S, Pillay M. High Reliability Organisation (HRO) Principles of Collective Mindfulness:

An Opportunity to Improve Construction Safety Management. In: Arezes P editor. Advances in Safety Management and Human Factors. AHFE 2018. Advances in Intelligent Systems and Computing. Vol. 791. Cham: Springer; 2019. DOI: 10.1007/978-3-319-94589-7_1

[17] Foisydoll L, Leighton K. Simulation Champions. Fostering Courage, Caring, and Connection. 1st ed. Philadelphia: LWW, Wolters Kluwer; 2018

[18] Knowles MS. The Modern Practice of Adult Education: From Pedagogy to Andragogy. Englewood Cliffs, N.J.: Cambridge Adult Education; 1988

[19] Steinert Y. Faculty Development in the Health Professions: A Focus on Research and Practice. Dordrecht: Springer; 2014. pp. 1-442

[20] Husebo S, O'Regan S. Reflective practice and its role in simulation. Clinical Simulation In Nursing. 2015;**11**(8):368-375. DOI: 10.1016/j.ecns.2015.04.005

[21] INACSL standards committee. INACSL standards of best practice: Simulation SM Simulation design. Clinical Simulation in Nursing. 2016;**12**:S5-S12. http://dx.doi.org/10.1016/j.ecns

[22] Jackson A, Halstead J. National League for Nursing Commission for nursing education accreditation. Nurse Educator. 2016;**41**(6):303. DOI: 10.1097/NNE.0000000000000309

[23] SSH Accreditation Standards [Internet]. 2019. Available from: https://www.ssih.org/Credentialing/Accreditation/Full-Accreditation

[24] INACSL Standards [Internet]. 2019. Available from: https://www.inacsl.org/inacsl-standards-of-best-practice-simulation/

[25] Definition of Patient Safety by the WHO [Internet]. 2019. Available from: https://www.who.int/patientsafety/about/en/

[26] Chilean law of Patient Safety. [Internet]. 2019. Available from: http://www.leychile.cl/Navegar?idNorma=1039348

[27] Indications for Hand Hygiene [Internet]. 2019. Available from: https://www.who.int/gpsc/tools/Five_moments/es/

[28] Surgical safety pause. [Internet]. 2019. Available from: https://www.who.int/patientsafety/safesurgery/sssl_manual_spanish.pdf

[29] Makary MA, Daniel M. Medical error - the third leading cause of death in the US. BMJ. 2016;**353**:i2139. DOI: 10.1136/bmj.i2139

[30] Kohn LT, Corrigan JM, Donaldson MS. To Err Is Human: Building a Safer Health System. Washington, D.C: National Academy Press; 2006

[31] Gaba DM. Anaesthesiology as a model for patient safety in health care. BMJ. 2000;**320**(7237):785-788. DOI: 10.1136/bmj.320.7237.785

[32] Global Standards for the Education of Nurses and Midwives. [Internet]. 2019. Available from: https://www.who.int/hrh/nursing_midwifery/hrh_global_standards_education.pdf

[33] Escudero EAM, Dominguez K. Simulación clínica y seguridad del paciente. Scientia Medica. 2018;**28**(1)

[34] Rossi EG, Bellandi T, Picchi M, Baccetti S, Monechi MV, Vuono C, et al. Patient safety in complementary medicine through the application of clinical risk management in the public health system. Medicines (Basel). 2017;**4**(4):93. DOI: 10.3390/medicines4040093

[35] Learning from Error. [Internet]. 2019. Available from: https://www.who.int/patientsafety/activities/technical/vincristine_learning-from-error.pdf

[36] Rall M, Dieckmann P. Simulation and patient safety: The use of simulation to enhance patient safety on a systems level. Current Anaesthesia and Critical Care. 2005;**16**(5):273-281. DOI: 10.1016/j.cacc.2005.11.007

[37] Weinger MB, Gaba DM. Human factors engineering in patient safety. Anesthesiology: The Journal of the American Society of Anesthesiologists. 2014;**120**(4):801-806. DOI: 10.1097/ALN.0000000000000144

[38] Gaba DM. Crisis resource management and teamwork training in anaesthesia. British Journal of Anaesthesia. 2010;**105**(1):3-6. DOI: 10.1093/bja/aeq124

[39] Gaba DM, Fish KJ, Howard SK, Burden AR, Company WBS. Crisis Management in Anesthesiology. Philadelphia: Elsevier/Saunders; 2015

[40] Kardong-Edgren S. Is simulationist a word? Clinical Simulation In Nursing. 2013;**9**(12):e561. DOI: 10.1016/j.ecns.2013.10.001

[41] Harder N. Simulation and patient safety: Continuing to provide evidence. Clinical Simulation In Nursing. 2019;**29**:38-39. DOI: 10.1016/j.ecns.2019.03.006

[42] Posner GD, Clark ML, Grant VJ. Simulation in the clinical setting: Towards a standard lexicon. Advances in Simulation. 2017;**2**(1):15. DOI: 10.1186/s41077-017-0050-5

[43] Rollison S, Blessing R, Kuszajewski ML, Muckler VC. In situ simulation to improve management of in-hospital strokes: Unexpected challenges. Clinical Simulation in Nursing. 2018;**24**:30-34. DOI: 10.1016/j.ecns.2018.09.004

[44] Randmaa M, Mårtensson G, Leo Swenne C, Engström M. SBAR improves communication and safety climate and decreases incident reports due to communication errors in an anaesthetic clinic: A prospective intervention study. BMJ Open. 2014;**4**(1):e004268. DOI: 10.1136/bmjopen-2013-004268

[45] King H, Battles J, Baker D, Alonso A, Salas E, Webster J, et al. TeamSTEPPS: Team Strategies and Tools to Enhance Performance and Patient Safety; 2008

[46] Miller GE. The assessment of clinical skills/competence/performance. Academic Medicine. 1990;**65**(Suppl. 9): S63-S67

[47] Scalese R, Obeso V, Issenberg B. Simulation Technology for Skills Training and Competency Assessment in medical education. Journal of General Internal Medicine. 2008;**23**(Suppl. 1):46-49. DOI: 10.1007/s11606-007-0283-4

[48] Boulet JR, Murray DJ. Simulation-based assessment in anesthesiology: Requirements for practical implementation. Anesthesiology. 2010;**112**(4):1041-1052. DOI: 10.1097/ALN.0b013e3181cea265

[49] Huang GC, McSparron JI, Balk EM, Richards JB, Smith CC, Whelan JS, et al. Procedural instruction in invasive bedside procedures: A systematic review and meta-analysis of effective teaching approaches. BMJ Quality and Safety. 2016;**25**(4):281-294. DOI: 10.1136/bmjqs-2014-003518

[50] Ma IW, Brindle ME, Ronksley PE, Lorenzetti DL, Sauve RS, Ghali WA. Use of simulation-based education to improve outcomes of central venous catheterization: A systematic review and meta-analysis. Academic Medicine. 2011;**86**(9):1137-1147. DOI: 10.1097/ACM.0b013e318226a204

[51] Corvetto MA, Fuentes C, Araneda A, Achurra P, Miranda P, Viviani P, et al. Validation of the imperial college surgical assessment device for spinal anesthesia. BMC Anesthesiology. 2017;**17**(1):131. DOI: 10.1186/s12871-017-0422-3

[52] Aggarwal R, Dosis A, Bello F, Darzi A. Motion tracking systems for assessment of surgical skill. Surgical Endoscopy. 2007;**21**(2):339. DOI: 10.1007/s00464-005-0561-3

[53] Corvetto MA, Altermatt FR. Tracking motion devices as assessment tools in anesthesia procedures: Have we been using them well? CJEM. 2017;**19**(5):412-413. DOI: 10.1017/cem.2017.337

[54] Clinkard D, Holden M, Ungi T, Messenger D, Davison C, Fichtinger G, et al. The development and validation of hand motion analysis to evaluate competency in central line catheterization. Academic Emergency Medicine. 2015;**22**(2):212-218. DOI: 10.1111/acem.12590

[55] Higham H, Greig PR, Rutherford J, Vincent L, Young D, Vincent C. Observer-based tools for non-technical skills assessment in simulated and real clinical environments in healthcare: A systematic review. BMJ Quality and Safety. 2019;**28**(8):672-686. DOI: 10.1136/bmjqs-2018-008565

[56] Boet S, Etherington N, Larrigan S, Yin L, Khan H, Sullivan K, et al. Measuring the teamwork performance of teams in crisis situations: A systematic review of assessment tools and their measurement properties. BMJ Quality and Safety. 2019;**28**:327-337. DOI: 10.1136/bmjqs-2018-008260

[57] Cooper S, Cant R, Porter J, Sellick K, Somers G, Kinsman L, et al. Rating medical emergency teamwork performance: Development of the TEAM emergency assessment measure (TEAM). Resuscitation. 2010;**81**(4):446-452. DOI: 10.1016/j.resuscitation.2009.11.027

[58] Lamé G, Dixon-Woods M. Using clinical simulation to study how to improve quality and safety in healthcare. BMJ Simulation and Technology Enhanced Learning. 2018. DOI: 10.1136/bmjstel-2018-000370. [Published Online]

[59] Green M, Tariq R, Green P. Improving patient safety through simulation training in anesthesiology: Where are we? Anesthesiology Research and Practice. 2016;**2016**:4237523. DOI: 10.1155/2016/4237523

[60] Cook DA, Aj L, Garside S. Method and reporting quality in health professions education research: A systematic review. Medical Education. 2011;**45**(3):227-238. DOI: 10.1111/j.1365-2923.2010.03890

[61] Gordon M, Darbyshire D, Baker P. Non-technical skills training to enhance patient safety: A systematic review. Medical Education. 2012;**46**(11):1042-1054. DOI: 10.1111/j.1365-2923.2012.04343

[62] Zendejas B, Brydges R, Wang AT, Cook DA. Patient outcomes in simulation-based medical education: A systematic review. Journal of General Internal Medicine. 2013;**28**(8):1078-1089. DOI: 10.1007/s11606-012-2264-5

Section 2

Patient Safety

Chapter 3

Keeping Patients Safe: The Critical Role of Medical Error Recovery

Theresa A. Gaffney

Abstract

Two decades after the Institute of Medicine Report, To Err is Human: Building a Safer Health System illuminated the high number of preventable deaths and adverse events associated with health care, medical errors remain a top global concern. To date, resources have been focused on preventing medical errors; however, the importance of error recovery must not be overlooked. Medical errors cannot be fully eliminated from our health care system, yet many errors can be recovered thus preventing patient harm. This chapter will (1) define and describe the error recovery process, (2) discuss the role of health care providers in error recovery, (3) explore strategies that enhance and prohibit error recovery, and (4) analyze characteristics that influence error recovery. Given the importance of patient safety within the health care industry, health care professionals and organizations must focus on both error prevention and error recovery as a key strategy in keeping patients safe.

Keywords: medical errors, error recovery, near miss, patient safety, expertise, culture, leadership, workload, high reliability

1. Introduction

Four out of every 10 patients are harmed while receiving care; costing payers an average of $8000 per admission [1, 2]. Errors related to diagnosis, medication errors, and unsafe surgical procedures are most frequently reported [1]. Over the past two decades, numerous resources and attention have been devoted to preventing medical errors and adverse events. Yet, in complex, high-risk systems, eliminating errors is unrealistic [3]. Safety practices must incorporate both error prevention and error recovery strategies.

This chapter will focus on error recovery as a critical safety strategy. Topics discussed in this chapter include (1) the error recovery process, (2) the role of health care providers in error recovery, (3) strategies that enhance and prohibit error recovery, and (4) individual and organizational characteristics that influence error recovery.

2. Magnitude of medical errors

Health care harm is a top safety concern globally. Medical errors occur when actions (intended or unintended) fail to meet their desired outcome, an action is not completed as intended, or the wrong action is taken to achieve an aim [4, 5]. In other words, errors result from unintended consequences as well as when health care providers make the wrong decision. The Institute of Medicine's (IOM) seminal report *To Err is Human*, first alerted the health care community and the public to the widespread nature of deaths attributed to medical errors [6]. According to the IOM, 44,000 to 98,000 patient deaths were attributed to medical errors in the United States annually [4]. A decade later, Classen et al. estimated that the medical error rate among hospitalized Medicare beneficiaries was nearly four times that of the IOM estimate [7]. Over the past two decades, national efforts to reduce medical errors have led to some improvement. For example, hospital-acquired conditions (HACs) declined by nearly 1 million instances from 2014 to 2017 [8]. Despite these efforts, in 2019, the World Health Organization (WHO) reported that globally, four out of every 10 patients are harmed while receiving care and at least five patients die every minute as a result of medical errors [1]. Although the exact number of patient deaths attributed to medical errors remains debatable, preventable deaths and adverse events are a significant safety issue.

Research investigating the nature and impact of medical errors within the health care system began in earnest in the 1990s. Initially, human behavior, such as carelessness, poor motivation, and inattention, was blamed as the source of medical errors [6]. However, a shift away from the physiological and psychological limitations of humans and toward system error introduced new safety lessons from areas outside of the traditional health care arena [3, 6, 9]. Strategies adapted from safety-critical industries such as transportation, manufacturing, and aviation brought forward important gains in the fight to improve patient safety.

Aviation safety, for example, depends on managing errors, both through prevention and recovery [9]. In 1995, the US Secretary of Transportation challenged the aviation industry to meet the goal of zero accidents [10]. Interventions such as crew resource management training, checklists, and new technologies were introduced to address attitudes, behavior, and performance with the goal of improving aviation safety. Considerable efforts and resources were invested in the industry to limit opportunities for human error. However, human error is inevitable, particularly in complex, high-hazard organizations, and the goal of zero errors was unrealistic [3]. As a result, the aviation industry recognized the importance of error recovery and began training pilots to identify and remediate errors when they occurred [11].

Still, health care is focused on preventing medical errors, leaving behind important lessons in correcting errors to reduce adverse events. Health care historically equates errors with failure, and failure is unacceptable [12]. Thus, the notion of error management is not easily embraced. Error management involves understanding the nature and extent of errors, changing the conditions that create errors, identifying behaviors and actions that mitigate damage from errors, and training personnel in their use [9]. Error management incorporates two unique aspects [6]. The first aspect is prevention or limiting the incidence of errors. The second aspect is containing the damaging effects of errors, also referred to as error recovery. Error recovery is a highly valued strategy in safety programs outside of health care and is emerging as an important safety strategy in keeping patients safe [13].

3. Complexity

Health care systems are highly complex organizations, consisting of numerous interconnected components including the patients and their condition, the procedure, the team's expertise, the equipment design and use, and the workload [4]. Communication and the urgency in which decisions are made add further complexity to the system. Finally, these complex systems operate in highly variable environments that are impacted by regulatory, fiscal and social considerations.

High-reliability organizations (HROs) are organizations that operate in complex, high-hazard domains for extended periods without serious accidents or catastrophic failures [14]. HROs are not immune to errors and adverse events, instead, they are preoccupied with failure. Defining features of HROs include their heightened sense of vigilance and ability to anticipate and detect problems early in order to prevent adverse events. HROs have learned to make systems as tolerant as possible toward error [6]. Understanding error recovery can support health care organizations on the journey toward high reliability.

In safety-critical systems, error recovery is equally as important as error prevention, as it is often the last barrier of defense before a near miss becomes an adverse event [15]. Error recovery is highly valued in other industries outside of health care, yet it is just beginning to be recognized as an important safety strategy in health care [16]. Both error prevention and error recovery strategies are needed to make greater strides in improving patient safety.

4. Error recovery model

The Eindhoven Model of Near Miss Reporting has been used to explore and define error recovery in safety-critical industries [17]. Errors stem from technical, organizational or human factors that set off a chain reaction that could result in adverse events. When dangerous situations develop, systems are designed with automatic safety mechanisms to prevent negative consequences. In the case of high-risk situations however, automatic safety mechanisms are not always enough to resolve errors. In these instances, human intuition, expertise, and flexibility are needed to intervene and recover the error before harm occurs. If the error is recovered before harm occurs, this is defined as a near miss.

The Eindhoven model offers insight into error recovery processes in health care settings [15]. Henneman and Gawlinski adapted the Eindhoven model to create the Nursing Near-Miss model to better understand the mechanisms nurses use to recover errors at the point of care. In this model, bedside nurses are the final line of defense between a near miss and an adverse event. The researchers pointed out that surveillance is a key strategy nurses use to prevent developing incidents from becoming adverse events. A growing body of literature describes the ingenuity and adaptability of health care providers in recovering errors.

5. Error recovery process

Error recovery is a three-step sequential process incorporating (1) identification, (2) interruption and (3) correction [17–19]. First, an error must be detected. Error identification or detection is the process of knowing that an error occurred and may be triggered by a mismatch in an expected outcome. This step is aimed at making errors quickly apparent, thereby enabling recovery. Factors such as knowing the patient, players, plan of care, and the environment aid in identifying medical errors [16, 20, 21].

Interrupting an error is the second step in the error recovery process. In this step, participants attempt to understand how the error occurred, the level of importance, and potential countermeasures that may be necessary to return the situation to normal [20–23]. Health care providers interrupt errors using actions such as offering assistance, clarifying orders, and even verbally interrupting [16].

Perseverance is key to correcting errors, particularly when error identification or interruption was not successful [16]. In this step, the focus is on deploying countermeasures to avert the error and reducing patient harm [20–23]. Being physically present, reviewing or confirming the plan of care, and involving other experts or leaders are successful strategies in correcting errors [16]. The system returns to its' safe state and patient harm is averted when errors are successfully recovered [19]. If errors are not successfully recovered, adverse events and potentially catastrophic consequences may occur.

Health care providers rely on flexibility, ingenuity, surveillance, and clinical judgment in recovering errors [16]. Henneman et al. first recognized the importance of surveillance in the error recovery process [15, 20, 21, 24]. Surveillance involves the continuous acquisition, analysis, and synthesis of information from both an individual and organizational perspective. Surveilling the patient and the environment enables providers to recognize developing complications and intervene appropriately. In contrast, when surveillance is lacking dangerous events may develop. Clinical judgment integrates knowledge, skills, expertise, and reasoning to recognize and address potentially dangerous situations [16]. Finally, providers use creativity and flexibility when devising and choosing appropriate strategies to interrupt and correct errors.

Researchers have attempted to quantify the number of errors recovered by health care providers. An integrated review of the literature noted that the magnitude of error recovery among nurses varies from as much as 18 times per 1000 patient days among medical-surgical nurses to as many as two errors per shift among critical care nurses [16]. Perioperative nurses have been known to recover as many as 11 errors per surgical case [22]. Nurses commonly recover errors related to medication errors, mismanagement of aversive systems, mismanagement of coexisting health issues, and improper use of precaution techniques in invasive monitoring [25]. Nurses accept that errors occur and see error recovery as an ongoing part of their job [15]. They regularly identify, interrupt, and correct errors, yet this information is rarely collected and analyzed. Thus, the important role that nurses contribute to patient safety is often invisible [16].

In addition to nurses, others play key roles in error recovery. A growing body of literature has explored strategies pharmacists employ to recover errors [23, 26]. Emergency department pharmacists were found to recover, on average, 7.8 medication errors per 100 patients [26]. A study of error recovery in community pharmacies found that pharmacists recovered numerous e-prescribing errors daily [23]. Most errors were caught at the identification stage of the error recovery process by pharmacists and technicians using strategies such as double checks and highlighting information on the printed e-prescription. Consulting with other pharmacy team members, reviewing the patient's history, and consulting with patients were strategies used to interrupt medication errors. Finally, pharmacists and technicians contacted prescribers to correct medication errors.

Patients and families also contribute to identifying and interrupting medical errors. A study of families of hospitalized children attempted to quantify the number of errors recovered by families. Benjamin et al. reported that 8% more medical errors were identified and interrupted when families were actively engaged with the health care team during family-centered rounds [27]. Families questioned medication changes, scheduling issues, and adverse drug reactions. The literature supports the notion that patients and families are increasingly involved in early error detection [28]. An analysis of near misses in the National Health Service found many instances of family members reminding staff about lapsed arrangements, pointing out overlooked care plans, and insisting on tests. The literature indicates that patients frequently identify communication and coordination related problems that may lead to adverse events [29]. Key strategies enabling them to prevent adverse events were knowing the patient and plan of care. Patients and families should be encouraged to actively engage in the care process and speak up when concerns arise [28].

While there is no standardized approach to capturing the magnitude of medical errors, front-line providers, as well as patients and families, play critical roles in recovering errors. Patients and families contribute to ongoing surveillance through active engagement in the care process. Effective communication between health care team members, patients and families aids in identifying and interrupting medical errors. Flexibility, creativity, clinical judgment, and surveillance are key strategies enabling health care providers to correct errors.

6. Characteristics influencing error recovery

Health care organizations are striving toward resilience during turbulent times in which they continue to struggle with access, cost and quality issues. Providers are challenged to make intricate decisions in dynamic, fast-paced, complex environments under tight time constraints. Errors are likely to occur under such conditions. Individual characteristics and organizational structures and processes can either help or hinder error recovery.

6.1 Individual characteristics

Individual characteristics that influence error recovery include expertise and workload [16]. Experts, like non-experts, are not immune to errors. However, what is unique about experts, is that they can recover errors more quickly than non-experts [12]. Experts unconsciously organize knowledge into manageable chunks that allow them to access and use critical information when necessary [12, 16, 30–32]. Experts rely on past experiences to help them identify cues and recognize patterns. They are better able to synthesize explicit and tacit knowledge in meaningful ways as compared to non-experts. Experts separate critical and relevant information from irrelevant information. In the end, experts develop what is known as deep smarts, a special form of wisdom that incorporates social, emotional, formal, and experiential knowledge [32]. As clinicians develop deep smarts, they exhibit greater confidence, perform more efficiently, and achieve higher levels of performance.

In the health care arena, experts use a multi-dimensional approach to integrate clinical judgment with knowledge of the patient, environment, and plan of care that allows them to more readily recover errors [16, 20, 21, 31]. A laboratory study of attending critical care physicians, residents, and medical students exploring the relationship between expertise and error recovery found that experts (physicians) recovered more (75%) errors than residents (61%) [33]. A study exploring the ability of dialysis nurses to recover errors determined that expert nurses detected more errors than non-expert nurses [34]. A study exploring error recovery among medical-surgical nurses found that expert nurses were four times more likely to recover medical errors than non-expert nurses [31].

Another hallmark of expertise is knowing when to deviate from standard protocols and employ shortcuts [35]. The ability to gauge tolerable risk in clinical situations is acquired over time and can only reside within experts. A study of trauma physicians and residents found that expert physicians made fewer errors when deviating from standard protocols than first- and second-year residents [31]. When deviations from standards or countermeasures are required to prevent adverse events the role of expertise should not be underestimated.

Workload is also associated with error recovery. When workload increases, nurses' ability to recover errors decreases [13, 31]. The notion of workload incorporates the demand placed on one's cognitive function, physical energy and the work pace itself [36]. Acute care settings are fast-paced, complex environments in which health care providers are constantly combining complex thinking processes with psychomotor and affective skills to deliver appropriate care and interventions [37]. Nurses, in particular, spend a great deal of time providing direct patient care and communicating with patients, families, and team members [38]. Patient care involves nursing process activities such as assessing patients' clinical conditions, judging the need for nursing care intervention, implementing nursing care measures, and evaluating the effects of therapy. Communication involves consulting with team members, delegating to others, and patient education. Nurses are forced to cognitively shifting between patients based on their condition, medications, therapies, and requests within tight timeframes. As stressors and demands build, the nurse's thought processes and attention are negatively affected. Error identification and interruption is a complex process that requires significant cognitive resources [39]. Consequently, when nurses are experiencing high cognitive loads, due to heavy patient assignments or workload, their cognitive defenses and capacity to recovery errors are diminished.

6.2 Organizational characteristics

In addition to individual characteristics that influence error recovery, there are organizational characteristics as well. These characteristics include a culture of safety and leadership.

A culture of safety is the most important organizational factor contributing to successful error recovery. Organizations with a strong culture of safety recover errors more readily [13, 16]. On average, there are 2.4 recovery opportunities per error [13]. When a recovery opportunity is missed, individuals and organizations have another opportunity to identify, interrupt and correct the error before harm occurs. Organizations that prioritize safety engage in practices and behaviors that enable ongoing surveillance and ultimately error recovery. Practices such as interdisciplinary bedside rounds, effective handoffs, reducing interruptions and facilitating open and ongoing communication enhance early identification and resolution of errors [20, 21, 27–29].

When organizations do not prioritize safety, errors are more likely to occur, and error recovery opportunities are missed. In this case, important safety checks are skipped, shortcomings in protocols and procedures are noted, and critical knowledge is not transferred between providers making it difficult for errors to be identified [13].

Supportive leadership is also an important organizational characteristic influencing error recovery. Studies noted that when all else fails, involving leadership in the final stage of error recovery is an effective countermeasure to prevent patient harm [20, 21, 31]. But the role of leadership goes well beyond stepping in as the voice of authority to recover errors. Financial constraints, time pressures, and performance constraints put additional strain on organizations and impact error recovery processes [36, 37]. Leadership must develop a portfolio of strategies aimed at managing errors that are coordinated between executives, middle management and frontline staff [40]. Middle managers can act as a buffer for front-line providers and negotiate for solutions to alleviate heavy workloads. Executives can ensure a culture of safety and prioritize safety over other domains when faced with competing pressures. Leadership decisions, at all levels, contribute to creating an environment that either facilitates or hinders error recovery at the point of care.

Organizations striving to consistently provide excellence in quality and safety for every patient, every time must make safety a priority. A key safety strategy in resilient organizations is early error detection and mitigation of medical errors [6].

This strategy must be embraced by the health care industry. Today, health care providers are making critical decisions in complex situations within tight time constraints which contribute to medical errors. When errors occur, expertise and workload are individual characteristics that enhance error recovery. Expertise must be retained and redeployed across the staff. Strategies to facilitate the transfer of expert knowledge or deep smarts to non-experts should be harnessed. Workload and staffing levels must facilitate error recovery. Thus, workload or care models that leverage expertise should be explored. Finally, systems and processes must be adapted to address the strengths and weaknesses of human cognitive functions, particularly as health care becomes more complex.

7. Conclusion

This chapter described the error recovery process, highlighted the role of health care providers in error recovery, identified strategies that enhance and prohibit error, and explored individual and organizational characteristics that influence error recovery. Health care providers, patients, and families demonstrated ingenuity and adaptability when recovering errors. Flexibility, creativity, surveillance, and clinical judgment of health care providers are key strategies in identifying, interrupting and correcting medical errors. Characteristics that enhance error recovery include individual provider expertise and organizational culture of safety. A burdensome workload is an organizational characteristic that inhibits error recovery.

The value of error recovery in keeping patients safe is clear, although undervalued in health care. Safety-critical industries recognize that errors cannot be fully eliminated and have embraced error recovery as a critical safety strategy. Health care must do the same.

8. Case study

Delivering chemotherapy to cancer patients is a high-risk activity with numerous opportunities for patient harm [41]. Although the incidence of medication errors in chemotherapy is low, the margin of error for administering toxic chemotherapeutic agents to cancer patients is very small. Memorial Sloan Kettering Cancer Center noticed that as the number of chemotherapy orders increased so too did the number of near-miss medication errors. To minimize medication errors, the hospital implemented the new role of a verification nurse (VN) to review all chemotherapy orders. If a discrepancy is noted in the chemotherapy order, VNs investigate the incident by referring to protocols, contacting the health care provider for clarification, referring to the patient's plan of care for updates or changes and maintaining open and ongoing communication with the team members. Evaluation of the new role noted a direct correlation between an increase in chemotherapy orders and patient volume with error recovery by VNs. While additional complexity added to an increased number of medical errors, the organization embraced the concept of error recovery. This is an example of how one hospital heightened their sense of vigilance and supported strategies to enable health care providers to anticipate and detect problems early to prevent adverse events.

Conflict of interest

The author has no real or perceived conflicts of interest.

Author details

Theresa A. Gaffney
Marymount University, Arlington, Virginia, USA

*Address all correspondence to: tgaffney@marymount.edu

References

[1] World Health Organization. WHO calls for urgent action to reduce patient harm in healthcare [Internet]. 2019. Available from: https://www.who.int/news-room/detail/13-09-2019-who-calls-for-urgent-action-to-reduce-patient-harm-in-healthcare [Accessed: 08 November 2019]

[2] The Betsy Lehman Center for Patient Safety. The financial and human cost of medical error [Internet]. 2019. Available from: https://betsylehmancenterma.gov/assets/uploads/Cost-of-Medical-Error-Report-2019.pdf [Accessed: 08 November 2019]

[3] Carthey J, de Leval M, Reason J. Institutional resilience in healthcare systems. BMJ Quality and Safety. 2001;**10**:29-32. DOI: 10.1136/qhc.10.1.29

[4] Leape L. A systems analysis approach to medical error. Journal of Evaluation in Clinical Practice. 1997;**3**:213-222

[5] Reason J. Human error: Models and management. BMJ (Clinical Research Ed.). 2000;**7237**:768-770

[6] Institute of Medicine (U.S.). To Err Is Human: Building a Safer Health System. Washington: National Academies Press; 2000

[7] Classen D, Resar R, Griffin F, Frederico F, Frankel T, Kimmel N, et al. Global "trigger tool" shows that adverse events in hospitals may be ten times greater than previously measured. Health Affairs. 2011;**30**:581-589. DOI: 10.1377/hlthaff.2011.0190

[8] Agency for Healthcare Research and Quality. AHRQ analysis finds hospital-acquired conditions declined by nearly 1 million from 2014-2017 [Internet]. 2019. Available from: https://www.ahrq.gov/news/newsroom/press-releases/hac-rates-declined.html [Accessed: 08 November 2019]

[9] Helmreich R. On error management: Lessons from aviation. BMJ. 2000;**320**: 781-785

[10] Latorella K, Prabhu P. A review of human error in aviation maintenance and inspection. International Journal of Industrial Ergonomics. 2000;**26**:133-161

[11] Airbus. Management flight operations briefing notes [Internet]. Available from: http://www.smartcockpit.com/docs/Error_Management.pdf [Accessed: 08 November 2019]

[12] Patel V. Failure to detect medical error [Internet]. 2010. Available from: https://www.youtube.com/watch?v=jkIrFxDBqKk [Accessed: 08 November 2019]

[13] Habraken MP, van der Schaaf TW. If only....: Failed, missed and absent error recovery opportunities in medication errors. Quality & Safety in Health Care. 2010;**1**:37-41. DOI: 10.1136/qshc.2007.026187

[14] Agency for Healthcare Research and Quality. High reliability [Internet]. 2019. Available from: https://www.psnet.ahrq.gov/primer/high-reliability [Accessed: 07 November 2019]

[15] Henneman EA, Gawlinski A. A "near-miss" model for describing the nurse's role in the recovery of medical errors. Journal of Professional Nursing. 2004;**3**:196-201

[16] Gaffney T, Hatcher B, Milligan R. Nurses' role in medical error recovery: An integrative review. Journal of Clinical Nursing. 2016;**25**:906-917. DOI: 10.111/jocn.13126

[17] van der Schaaf TW. Near miss reporting in the chemical process industry: An overview. Microelectronics and Reliability. 1995;**9-10**:1233-1243. DOI: 10.1016/0026-2714(95)99374-R

[18] Kessels-Habraken M, van der Schaaf TW, de Jong J, Rutte C. Defining near misses: Toward a sharpened definition based on empirical data about error handling processes. Social Science & Medicine. 2010;**70**:1301-1308

[19] van der Schaaf TW, Kanse L. Errors and Error Recovery. In: Elzer PF, Kluwe RH, Boussoffara B, editors. Human Error and System Design and Management. Godalming: Springer; 2000

[20] Henneman EA, Blank F, Gawlinski A, Henneman P. Strategies used by nurses to recover medical errors in an academic emergency department setting. Applied Nursing Research. 2006;**2**:70-77

[21] Henneman EA, Gawlinski A, Blank F, Henneman P, Jordan D. MKJ. Strategies used by critical care nurses to identify, interrupt, and correct medical errors. American Journal of Critical Care. 2010;**6**:500-509. DOI: 10.4037/ajcc2010167

[22] Yang Y, Henry L, Dellinger M, Yonish K, Emerson B, Seifert PC. The circulating nurse's role in error recovery in the cardiovascular OR. AORN Journal. 2012;**6**:755-762

[23] Odukoya O, Stone J, Chiu M. How do community pharmacies recover from e-prescription errors? Research in Social & Administrative Pharmacy. 2014;**10**:837-852. DOI: 10.1016/j.sapharm.2013.11.009

[24] Henneman EA. Recognizing the ordinary as extraordinary: Insight into the "way we work" to improve patient safety. American Journal of Critical Care. 2017;**26**:272-276. DOI: 10.4037/ajcc2017812

[25] Dykes PC, Rothschild JM, Hurley AC. Medical errors recovered by critical care nurses. The Journal of Nursing Administration. 2010;**5**:241-246

[26] Rothschild J, Churchill W, Erickson A, Munz K, Schuur JD, Salzberg CA, et al. Medication errors recovered by emergency department pharmacists. Annals of Emergency Medicine. 2010;**55**:513-521. DOI: 10.1016/j.annemergmed.2009.10.012

[27] Benjamin J, Cox E, Trapskin P, Rajamanickam V, Jorgenson R, Weber H, et al. Family-initiated dialogue about medications during family-centered rounds. Pediatrics. 2015;**1**:135-194. DOI: 10.1542/peds.2013-3885

[28] Lang S, Garrido MV, Heintze C. Patients' view of adverse events in primary and ambulatory care: A systematic review to assess methods and the content of what patients consider to be adverse events. BMC Family Practice. 2016;**17**. DOI: 10.1186/s12875-016-0408-0

[29] Gillespie A, Reader T. Patient-centered insights: Using healthcare complaints to reveal hotspots and blindspots in quality and safety. The Milbank Quarterly. 2018;**96**(3):530-567. DOI: 10.1111/1468-0009.12338

[30] Ambrose S, Bridges M, DiPietro M, Lovett M, Norman M. How Learning Works. San Francisco CA: Jossey-Bass; 2010

[31] Gaffney T, Hatcher B, Milligan R, Trickey A. Enhancing patient safety: Factors influencing medical error recovery among medical-surgical nurses. Online Journal of Issues in Nursing. 2016;**23**(3):1-12

[32] Leonard D, Swap W. Deep Smarts. Boston: Harvard School Press; 2005

[33] Patel VL, Cohen T, Murarka T, Olsen J, Kagita S, Myneni S, et al. Recovery at the edge of error: Debunking the myth of the infallible expert. Journal of Biomedical Informatics. 2011;**44**:413-424

[34] Wilkinson W, Cauble L, Patel V. Error detection and recovery in dialysis nursing. Journal of Patient Safety. 2011;**7**:213-223

[35] Kahol K, Vankipuram M, Patel VL, Smith ML. Deviations from protocol in a complex trauma environment: Errors or innovations. Journal of Biomedical Informatics. 2011;**44**:425-431. DOI: 10.1016/j.jbi.2011.04.003

[36] Guastello S, Correro A, Marra D. Cusp catastrophe models for cognitive workload and fatigue in teams. Applied Ergonomics. 2019;**79**:152-168. DOI: 10.1016/j.apergo.2018.08.019

[37] Redding D, Robinson S. Interruptions and geographic challenges to nurses' cognitive workload. Journal of Nursing Care Quality. 2009;**24**(3):194-200

[38] Potter P, Wolf L, Boxerman S, Grayson D, Sledge J, Dunagan C, et al. An analysis of nurses' cognitive work: A new perspective for understanding medical error. In: Henriksen K, Battles JB, Marks ES, et al, editors. Advances in Patient Safety: From Research to Implementation. Vol. 1. Washington, DC: Agency for Healthcare Research and Quality (US); 2005. pp. 39-51

[39] Patel V, Kannampallil T, Shortliffe E. Role of cognition in generating and mitigating clinical errors. BMJ Quality and Safety. 2015;**24**:468-474. DOI: 10.1136/bmjqs-2014-003482

[40] Amalberti R, Vincent C. Managing risk in hazardous conditions: Improvisation is not enough. BMJ Quality and Safety. 2020;**29**:60-63. DOI: 10.1136/ bmjqs-2019-009443

[41] Baldwin A, Rodriguez E. Improving patient safety with error identification in chemotherapy orders by verification nurses. Clinical Journal of Oncology Nursing. 2016;**20**(1):59-66. DOI: 10.1188/16.CJON.59-65

Chapter 4

Patient Safety in a First-Level Hospital in Colombia, According to London Protocol

Carmen Luisa Betancur Pulgarín,
Mónica Roció Romero Carvajal, Luis Gabriel Murillo Micolta,
Yaqueline Churi Antero, Yudi Nathalia Angulo Ante
and Diego Carmona Carmona

Abstract

The objective of this study is to identify the adherence of the health personnel of the state social enterprise Norte 2 institution, Caloto, Department of Cauca, Colombia, in the application of the London protocol, referring to patient safety policy, where a quantitative investigation was conducted; observational, descriptive through a census of 92 officials of the institution through a survey designed to measure adherence to protocol, all information was tabulated in the Epi-info 7.2 program and presented by descriptive statistics; the results of this study showed that the population is composed of 60% of female nursing assistants who are more than 1-year old and that the protocol is partially met, where it was found that only 52% of adverse events are reported, concluding that there is no defined patient safety culture, which means that adverse events are not documented.

Keywords: MeSH and DeCS, adverse event, preventable adverse event, Non-preventable adverse event, London protocol, patient safety policy

1. Introduction

Health care over time has become a complex and very careful act, which, in addition to providing users with adequate treatment for their health problems, represents a latent risk since it can cause involuntary damage. This, for obvious reasons, since 2002 the World Health Organization (WHO), requested in Resolution WHA55.18 the member states to pay as much attention as possible to the problem of patient safety [1]. This difficulty being an attenuator over time has become a public health problem that directly impacts the quality of care of users of health services and the fall in their indicators.

This World Alliance, which aims to coordinate, disseminate, and accelerate the improvement of patient safety worldwide, is a means that fosters international collaboration and the adoption of measures among member states, the WHO secretariat, the technical experts and consumers, professionals, and industrial groups [2]. Different studies conducted in our country at different levels of care, such as the ENEAS study, the National Study on Adverse Effects linked to Hospitalization [3], and the Study on Patient Safety in Primary Health Care (APEAS) [4], have quantified the importance of these effects.

Different investigations have been found in relation to patient safety, where the one carried out by Villareal [5] is found, in Third World countries and in those with transition economy; there is evidence that the probability in the occurrence of adverse events is caused due to the poor state of the infrastructure and the equipment, the quality of the medicines, the irregularity in the supply, the deficiency in waste disposal and infection control, and the poor performance of the staff due to lack of motivation or knowledge is insufficient and due to the serious lack of resources to cover essential operating costs.

Also in 2011, Blandón, Gómez, Muñoz, and Zafra [6] carried out a patient safety audit process from the analysis of the adverse event report at the Francisco Luís Jiménez Martínez de Carepa hospital (Antioquia), where flaws were evident in the fulfillment of the processes related to the prevention of events and where improvement activities were proposed in order to minimize and prevent the recurrence of events highlighting the awareness of all personnel prioritizing those who work in the emergency department on adverse events, in addition to developing improvement plans regarding the control of dangerous conditions in the physical environment.

In 2013, an investigation was conducted on safety culture and adverse events in a first-level clinic [7]; this shows the prevalence of adverse events in nursing staff, where the main errors were the lack of communication and techniques of poor application of medications in nursing staff which affects patients in 29.9% producing an adverse event. In 2014 Meléndez Concepción, Garza, González, Castillo, González, and Hernández [8] conducted an investigation on the perception of nurses towards the culture of safety in a pediatric hospital in Mexico, where the average age of the respondents was 49 years old for men, 91% were women, and 70% were general nurses. Nurses believe that the strengths that are available in the hospital are few and that many things are missing to ensure patient safety.

Poma Vanessa [9] developed an investigation with the purpose of contributing to the improvement of quality and safety in the care of patients of the internal medicine service of the Eugenio mirror hospital in the city of Quito, in 2015, for which it was carried out a parallel between the reality evidenced in the service and the national and international quality standards of process and results structure where it could be established that the institution did not meet the specific criteria in terms of structure and results compared to international standards, so which emphasized the safety culture of internal users as well as of patients as a fundamental axis for continuous improvement, revealing not only the failures of the institution but also the responsibility of the collaborators of the institution.

In the IBEAS study, Colombia specifically showed a prevalence of adverse events of 13.1%, 27.3% of the events occurred in children under 15 years, and 27.7% occurred during the performance of a procedure [10] and where it has been estimated by WHO under its studies that one in 10 hospitalized patients suffers an incident that will cause damage during their stay. Studied in countries with medium and high economies, is not yet known in countries with emerging economies, but it is thought that in these, the magnitude of the problem may be even greater [11], which allows to demonstrate that in general terms, health in Colombia is going through a difficult stage in terms of quality.

For its part, the state social enterprise Norte 2 located in the municipality of Caloto, department of Cauca, is a social enterprise of the state that provides health care of low complexity for around 7000 people living in the municipality. This institution as a company that currently provides health services has found that the patient safety protocol established by the Ministry of Health and Social Protection is not being applied under the guidelines of the patient safety policy in Resolution 0112 of 2012. In addition to this, health professionals for unknown reasons do not apply the London protocol and generally do not exercise the functions of inspection, surveillance, and control in order to provide reports in a timely manner, to take corrective actions and relevant improvement to mitigate adverse events that are becoming increasingly evident.

The objective of the present investigation is to identify the adherence of the health personnel of the state social enterprise Norte 2 health institution, Caloto, Cauca, during the first quarter of 2019, in the application of the London protocol, referring to the security policy of the patient, to propose an improvement plan according to the results obtained. In this sense, the application of the London protocol in patient safety policy in the state social enterprise Norte 2 health institution is of vital importance, in order to impact on the improvement of the quality of health care as a systematic tool for a continuous improvement defined in the mandatory quality assurance system, increasing its quality of service making it a competitive entity.

In Colombia, the Ministry of Health and Social Protection [12] defines patient safety as the set of structural elements, processes, instruments, and methodologies based on scientifically proven evidence that tend to minimize the risk of suffering, an adverse event in the process of health care or mitigate its consequences. Under the obligatory system of quality assurance of health care, the country, through its components, seeks and promotes a patient safety policy whose objective is to prevent the occurrence of situations that affect patient safety and reduce and if possible eliminate the occurrence of adverse events to have safe and competitive institutions internationally [13].

In addition to this, Resolution 2003 of 2014 [14] dictates the design of processes and procedures focused on the promotion of safe health care, the identification of the risks in health care provided to patients in different services and its prioritization and intervention, the definition of safe care processes, the education of patients and their families in the knowledge and approach of the factors that can influence in improving the safety of the care processes of which they are subjected, and the application of mandatory safe practices, reporting, measurement, analysis, and management of adverse events.

More than a concept, it is a movement that emerges worldwide as a rethinking of the effectiveness of health systems in different countries. Health systems and especially the professionals that integrate it, without a doubt, aim at the well-being of patients; however, despite their good intentions, they can also cause harm [15]. The effectiveness of health systems then depends not only on the impact caused by the improvement of the health of the users but also on the safety conditions in which care is given, which is the raison d'être of the patient's safety policy: provide safe and effective care.

According to the Ministry of Social Action [16], the guidelines of the London protocol are taken under the guiding principles of the policy in order to achieve the purpose of establishing safe attention; it goes beyond the establishment of standards; these are only the frame of reference. The commitment and cooperation of the different actors is necessary to raise awareness and promote, arrange, and coordinate actions that really achieve effective achievements. Patient safety problems are inherent in health care. For this purpose it is relevant to establish transversal principles that guide all the actions to be implemented.

Patient safety is presented as a fundamental pillar within the patient safety protocol, which is defined as the set of organizational structures or processes that reduce the probability of adverse events resulting from exposure to the care system. Have medical attention throughout the procedures or diseases [17]. In this way, patient safety is part of a whole set of legal requirements, which must be fully complied with by health professionals, which guarantee that the patient is prevented from any risk present in medical services.

In this regard and under the London protocol in patient safety policy, according to the Ministry of Social Action [18], the guidelines of the London protocol are taken. The guiding principles of the policy are that achieving the purpose of establishing safe attention goes beyond the establishment of standards; these are only the frame of reference. The commitment and cooperation of the different actors is necessary to raise awareness and promote, arrange, and coordinate actions that really achieve effective achievements. Patient safety problems are inherent in health care. For this purpose, it is relevant to establish transversal principles that guide all the actions to be implemented [19]. These principles are as follows:

1. User-centered focus of attention. It means that the important thing is the results obtained in it and its safety, which is the axis around which all the patient's safety actions revolve.

2. Security culture. The environment for the deployment of patient safety actions must take place in an environment of confidentiality and trust between patients, professionals, insurers, and the community. It is the duty of the different actors of the system to facilitate the conditions that allow the said environment.

3. Integration with the mandatory quality assurance system of health care. The patient safety policy is an integral part of the mandatory quality assurance system of health care and is transversal to all its components.

4. Multicausality. The problem of patient safety is a systemic and multicausal problem in which different organizational areas and different actors must be involved [20].

Under the conceptual model and basic definitions of patient safety policy, the following figure shows in a pictorial way the conceptual model on which the terminology used in this document is based, and then the definitions related to the different items raised and used are included in the patient safety policy of the compulsory quality assurance system of health care. It is necessary to integrate international terminology with specificities of the terminology requirements identified in the country [21].

The methods used were designed with the aim of promoting an open environment that contrasts with the traditional ones based on personal accusations and fault allocation. This protocol covers the process of research, analysis, and recommendations. There is no need to insist that the proposed methodology has to be separated, as far as possible, from disciplinary procedures and those designed to address permanent individual poor performance. In health, very often when something goes wrong, bosses tend to overestimate the contribution of one or two individuals and assign them to blame for what happened [22].

This does not mean that the indictment cannot exist, what it means is that this should not be the starting point, among other things, because the immediate allocation of guilt distorts and hinders subsequent serious and thoughtful investigation. Effectively reducing the risks implies taking into account all the factors, changing the environment and dealing with the failures by action or omission of the people. This is never possible in an organization whose culture puts disciplinary considerations first. In order for incident investigation to be fruitful, it must be carried out in an open and fair environment [22].

For its part, the organizational model of causality of clinical incidents is supported under the theory of the protocol, and its applications are based on research conducted outside the field of health. In aviation and in the oil and nuclear industries, accident investigation is an established routine. Safety specialists have developed a wide variety of methods of analysis, some of which have been adapted for use in clinical care contexts [23].

In this way, they raise the need to conduct the investigation and analysis of incidents (errors or adverse events), which refer to the basic process of investigation and analysis is quite standardized. It was designed with the idea that it is useful and can be used both in minor incidents and in serious adverse events. It does not change if it is executed by a person or a large team of experts. In the same way, the investigator (person or team) can decide how fast he goes through it, from a short session to a full investigation that can take several weeks, including a thorough examination of the chronology of the facts, of the unsafe actions, and of the contributory factors. The decision about the length and depth of the investigation depends on the severity of the incident, the resources available, and the potential institutional learning [24].

And where under the Reason model of causality (Swiss cheese model), belonging to the problem solving and identification models, it works to identify what aspects or decisions of the organization may have been a conditioning factor in an accident and how the organization can learn from an accident, perfecting the defenses in a cycle of continuous improvement [25, 26]. Also called Swiss cheese model, which was raised in order to analyze the possible causes that develop potential risks, the model compares the causes of risk with layers of Swiss cheese, where for an action to be generated, several failures are required to reach this, since, if there is a barrier, that potential cause will undoubtedly not allow it to become damage. It speaks of four factors that contribute to the extent of the damage: insufficient training, poor communication, lack of supervision, and inadequate apparatus [27].

On the issue of safety, the causes identified have been grouped in different ways (organizational causes, equipment, supplies, people, etc.) and specifically on the issue of patient safety. In the United Kingdom, an organizational model for the causality of errors and adverse events (organizational accident causation model) was developed in the context of the so-called London protocol or "systems analysis of clinical incidents—the London protocol" [28, 29]. Among the possible solutions is the fishbone formulated by Ishikawa who was an industrial chemist and a business administrator, in response to the need to implement quality in business processes and services. Through its proposal it is easy to observe the relationship between cause and effect. Mention six components that lead to the problem which are labor, material, method, machine, measuring, and environment [30].

2. Materials and methods

This research is quantitative, observational, and descriptive, and a census was carried out on the 92 officials of the state social enterprise Norte 2, Caloto, Cauca (Colombia, Sur America) institution, under the inclusion criteria: be a worker linked to the institution by employment contract, have the institutional consent of the company, and have informed and understood consent with each of the units of analysis and where exclusion criteria are not contemplated. Study variables such as sociodemographic characteristics, knowledge variables, and improvement variables were taken into account.

The analysis plan of the present investigation had the collection of information through a survey created by the researchers and reviewed by four experts in the field; for the tabulation of the data, the researchers created an instrument to obtain a database in the Epiinfo 7.2 program; this program is a free epidemiological analysis software supplied by the World Health Organization and in which the analysis of results with descriptive statistics was performed. The bioethical component was aligned in accordance with Resolution 008430 of 1993 and Resolution 0314 of 2018 which regulates ethical responsibilities in research in humans and health institutions, taking into account that the research has a lower risk than the minimum. Complying with Colombian regulations, institutional consent and informed consent were obtained by each participant. The credits of the institution in which the research is carried out are included, according to copyright.

For research the guidelines of the London protocol are taken. The guiding principles of the policy with which, to achieve the purpose of establishing safe attention, goes beyond setting standards; these are only the frame of reference. The commitment and cooperation of the different actors is necessary to raise awareness, promote, arrange, and coordinate actions that really achieve effective achievements. Patient safety problems are inherent in health care. The transversal principles that guide the actions to be implemented are:

1. User-centered focus of attention. It means that the important thing is the results obtained in it and its safety, which is the axis around which all the patient's safety actions revolve.

2. Security culture. The environment for the deployment of patient safety actions must take place in an environment of confidentiality and trust between patients, professionals, insurers, and the community. It is the duty of the different actors of the system to facilitate the conditions that allow the said environment.

3. Integration with the mandatory quality assurance system of health care. The patient safety policy is an integral part of the mandatory quality assurance system of health care and is transversal to all its components.

4. Multicausality. The problem of patient safety is a systemic and multicausal problem in which different organizational areas and different actors must be involved.

An instrument with 12 specific questions about patient safety and questions about demographic aspects was implemented. The specific questions, with multiple answer options, and yes or no, were:

1. What is the definition of adverse event?

2. Do you know the protocol model for the report of adverse events?

3. Have you received trainings from the institution in protocols that guarantee patient safety?

4. Does the institution have the patient safety program to obtain safer care processes? Do you know?

5. In case of an adverse event, would you ask for support for report?

6. Who is the official in charge of performing the report of the adverse event?

7. What is the main cause why you do not report the adverse events?

8. Do you notify all reports of adverse events, clinical incidents, and complications related to health care?

9. What do you consider is the main cause for not reporting adverse events related to health care?

10. What is the definition of clinical incident?

11. What is the definition of clinical complication?

12. Does the institution perform the feedback of adverse events?

3. Results

It was found that demographically the female gender represents more than half of the population, being mostly people with a technical academic level, who have been in ESE for more than a year, and of which three out of four are auxiliary of nursing, which represents a population trained in technical tasks linked to day-to-day work in the ESE, with an experience of more than 1 year within the said institution in three out of four officials; on the other hand, it is observed that only 1 of every 11 people in the population are nurses, who are in charge of coordinating these assistants and are the guarantors of the proper performance of all protocols within the institution (**Table 1**).

For the frequency of response according to the definition of adverse events according to the London protocol, it is possible to justify that the entire population surveyed is clear about the concept of the definition of adverse events under current regulations, which demonstrates that the ESE performs an adequate accompaniment regarding the acquisition of knowledge regarding the definitions of the terminology used within its facilities, which allows all its collaborators to be in the same tuning, avoiding communication problems in terms of technical terminology and knowledge of the laws and resolutions of the ministry of health that define under presidential ruling the conception of these.

For the knowledge of the London protocol model for the reporting of adverse events, officials have one out of five present ignorance of the protocol, which can lead

Variable	Answer	Frequency	Percentage
Sex	Female	61	66
	Male	31	34
Education level	Technical	67	73
	Professional	14	15
	Support	6	7
	Others	5	5
Antiquity	Under one year	29	32
	Older than one year	63	68
Job that performs	Doctor	4	4
	Nurse	6	7
	Dentist	3	3
	Nursing assistant	64	70
	Other	15	16

Table 1.
Frequency of demographic variables of health personnel of state social enterprise Norte 2, Caloto, Cauca, Colombia, in the first half of 2019.

to failures in the practice of this, either due to lack of training and induction or recognition and omission which generates a latent risk both in terms of the quality of the service provided and in the care provided to the patient, putting his integrity at risk. In addition to the frequency in terms of training carried out by staff in the institution in protocols that guarantee patient safety, there is a group of people who have not received training in the patient safety protocol, which is presented as an administrative failure on the part of the institution, and the area in charge of carrying out the training of the collaborators, 1 of every remaining 11 has omitted the training provided by the ESE, generating problems that directly compromise patients and their safety.

The institution has the patient safety program to obtain safer care processes. Less than half of the respondents acknowledge that the institution has the patient safety program in terms of obtaining safer care processes, this amount being less than half of the officials surveyed, which describes a total lack of awareness for more than half of these, which generates a critical picture given that ignorance is counterproductive, given the nature of the ESE, demonstrating that more socialization of the documentation that the institution possesses, as well as training and documentation, is needed of the programs.

When an adverse event occurs, who is the person in charge of supporting the report of an adverse event? According to the established protocol, it was found that the person in charge of supporting the report of an adverse event is intended to guarantee quality of health care and serve as a bridge to generate a solution to the event presented; in this sense there is no consensus, given the ignorance of the protocol and the poor socialization of this both by the administrative area and by the same care staff, where more than half of the officials have full knowledge of who is the person in charge of carrying out the accompaniment and providing support if necessary when an adverse event occurs.

Likewise, within the knowledge of the official responsible for making the report of the adverse event according to the established protocol, it is described that within the report of the adverse event, the immediacy in the realization of this has its incidence within the quality system and of the patient safety protocol; for this reason the person who detects the adverse event must perform it in a short period of time when it is detected; in this sense more than half of the respondents know who should do it, with which you can affirm that some of these seek to separate themselves from their functions or they are not aware of the protocol and the step by step to follow when an event of these occurs, looking for a way to lighten your workload, **Figure 1**.

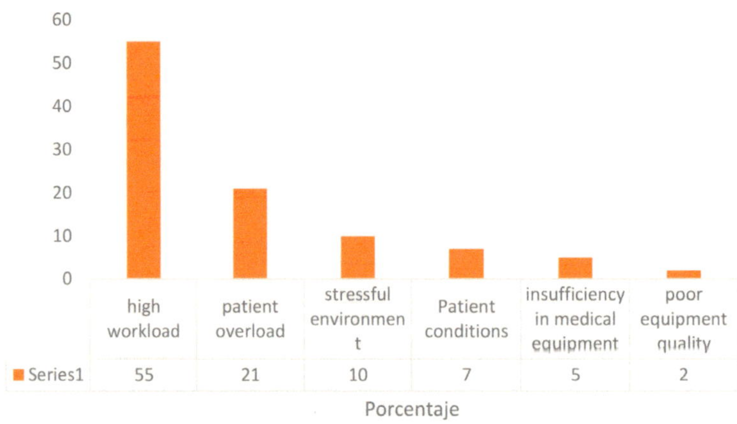

Figure 1.
Main cause for not reporting adverse events related to health care.

The frequency of response regarding the most frequent cause of not reporting adverse events, it was found that the main causes of failure to report adverse events are divided perceptions, since on average 3 of every 11 believe that the mistakes made within their daily work will be a cause for dismissal, which shows the lack of knowledge of the internal regulations of the institution regarding the grounds for withdrawal, and a similar average thinks that the they have used it during their rest or active breaks, which is linked to another portion, which states that the workload does not allow their report, which must be reported immediately after its occurrence, as evidenced by the ignorance of both its functions and the patient safety protocol.

Within the culture of patient safety, the reporting of adverse events, clinical incidents, and related complications in health care allows the generation of corrective and improvement actions within the health system, which by not reporting or reporting spontaneously, like 4 out of 11 of the officials surveyed, it does not allow for the maturation or improvement of this, since the causes for which adverse events are being generated are unknown and opportunities for the quality team to solve underlying problems are lost. In this sense, a percentage close to half of the respondents duly report the adverse events and other incidents and complications, this being a lack of empowerment by the collaborator who does not have a safety culture present in their work.

The most frequent cause of not reporting adverse events related to health care, evidence within the different research questions, that the workload prevails, in this sense in more than half being the main cause for not reporting an adverse event, this situation being an attenuating one, since it is possible to relate directly to the lack of human resources within the institution, or the charges within it are not level with the staff, which is supported by two out of ten who affirm that the overload of patients also does not allow an adverse event to be reported, missing opportunities for improvement within the institution that manage to generate a positive effect within the care of patients.

For the frequency of response for the definition of clinical incident according to the London protocol, it can be affirmed that within the theoretical knowledge of ESE officials, it is found that more than half of the respondents know the definition of clinical incident, and a small part present difficulties in answering correctly, this being a serious failure, when making the report of an adverse event, since the misrepresentation of the terms can cause misunderstandings and that at the time of generating a report, the indicators are erroneous regarding the nature of adverse events. However, for the definition of clinical complication, approximately four out of every five officials know its concept, which shows that only a considerable minority represents confusion, which, in a real plane, can generate confusion and ignorance of the steps to follow or perform incorrect procedures, since the nature of each event is different and must be known from the theoretical basis in order to be clear about the concepts.

Within the administrative failures found, the socialization of adverse events in the institution, only half of these are carried out, which demonstrates that the commitment that exists within the protocol is not adequate within the nature of this; there is also one in five people who do not know if they do it or not, which allows us to affirm that there is a problem of latent communication within the ESE and the collaborators; they do not know everything, given the different shifts they have and the changes in the staff schedules, as well as their lack of commitment to the quality system of the institution, being a very marked problem within the institution, seeking to improve this perception within the collaborators.

4. Discussion

After the analysis of the results, investigations found that, under the same study theme, they manage to show similar results regarding the patient's safety policy and what was found in state social enterprise Norte 2 of Caloto, Cauca. It was found in the study carried out by Villareal [15] that the results obtained show that the institutions of Third World countries such as Colombia do not fully meet certain requirements for the reduction of adverse events, taking into account variables such as infrastructure, the state of the equipment, the quality and adequate supply of medicines, and the motivation of the staff, which confirms what was found in state social enterprise Norte 2, where professional and care personnel do not have full knowledge of the policies, in addition there was little motivation given the high workload they maintain and the low culture of patient safety that exists.

In 2014, Meléndez, Concepción, Garza, González, Castillo, González, and Hernández [19] found that within the demographic variables, the care staff has an age greater than 6 months, and where the average age of the respondents was 49 years, 91% were women and 70% are general nurses, who presented adherence to the patient safety protocol, which differs from what was found in the state social enterprise in Caloto, Cauca, since although the majority of the population were 69% women and nurses, older than 1 year, they did not show adherence to the humanization protocol of the patient due to different causes such as ignorance of the general concepts and the low report of adverse events.

Blandón, Gómez, Muñoz, and Zafra [16] carried out a security audit process that showed flaws in the fulfillment of the processes related to the prevention of events, where improvement activities were proposed in order to minimize and prevent the recurrence of events highlighting the awareness of all personnel, which corroborates what was found in the present investigation, since the staff does not comply with the safety culture regarding the reporting of adverse events, being necessary to propose actions which improves proposals, a plan prepared for them in order to reduce this problem.

In general, the research presented a difficulty which was access to primary information, and some of the professionals were reluctant to conduct the survey, as well as access to these for their work shifts was complicated, but nevertheless within the achievements, the latent problem was found in terms of both administrative and assistance failures of professionals, which do not present a culture of patient safety, and therefore, opportunities for improvement were found by creating a plan for improvement.

Converting the organizational culture for the improvement of the processes is one of the main objectives since adopting it as a culture will be immersed in the daily life of the institution, thus leading to continuous improvement reaching the expected quality. The contribution of reading about this program executed in the aforementioned institution serves as a guide and guidance that contributes to the enrichment of knowledge that allows the implementation of the audit plan to improve the quality of health care in the institution providing health services.

5. Conclusion

With the completion of the previous investigation, it is concluded that state social enterprise Norte 2, CALOTO CAUCA does not comply with the adherence to the London protocol in patient safety policy, taking into account that only 70% of officials It has adherence to this protocol, in addition, only 52% of adverse events are reported, the main cause of not being carried out, the workload and the little time they have for administrative work.

Conflicts of interest

The investigators do not declare conflicts of interest.

Thanks

We thank the institution state social enterprise Norte 2 Caloto, Cauca, manager, officials, quality team, and coordinating chiefs, who allowed our research team to be part of their institution to carry out our purpose and successfully complete the planned, and the University Foundation of the Andean area that were present to give us their support through their work team offering an education with excellence.

Author details

Carmen Luisa Betancur Pulgarín*, Mónica Roció Romero Carvajal*, Luis Gabriel Murillo Micolta*, Yaqueline Churi Antero*, Yudi Nathalia Angulo Ante* and Diego Carmona Carmona
Fundación Universitaria del Área Andina, Pereira, Colombia

*Address all correspondence to: calube@utp.edu.co, moromero@estudiantes.areandina.edu.co, lmurillo@estudiantes.areandina.edu.co, ychuri@estudiantes.areandina.edu.co and yangulo5@estudiantes.areandina.edu.co

References

[1] WHO. Patient Safety [Internet]. 2015. Disponible en: http://www.who.int/patientsafety/patients_for_patient/statement/es/ [citado 19 de noviembre 2018]

[2] Organización Mundial de la Salud. 59ª Asamblea Mundial de la Salud, Seguridad del Paciente. 2006. Disponible en: http://apps.who.int/gb/ebwha/pdf_files/WHA59-REC1/s/WHA59_2006_REC1-sp.pdf

[3] Aranaz J, Aibar C, Ruiz P. Estudio nacional sobre efectos adversos ligados a la hospitalización (ENEAS). Madrid: Ministerio de Sanidad y Consumo; 2005

[4] Estudio AJ, APEAS. Estudio sobre la seguridad de los pacientes en Atención Primaria de Salud. Madrid: Ministerio de Sanidad y Política Social; 2008

[5] Villareal E. Seguridad de los pacientes. Un compromiso de todos para un cuidado de calidad. Artículo de Reflexión. En: Salud Uninorte. 2017:23. Disponible en: http://www.redalyc.org/pdf/817/81723111.pdf

[6] Blandón G, Gómez M, Zafra E. Seguridad del paciente desde el análisis del reporte de evento adverso en la empresa social del estado hospital francisco Luís jiménez martínez de carepa, durante el año 2010, Apartado; 2011. Disponible en: http://repository.ces.edu.co/bitstream/10946/2429/2/TESIS%20CON%20LAS%20NORMAS%20ICONTEC%20_ULTIMO%20ENVIO_%5B2%5D.pdf

[7] Toffoletto M, Ramírez X. Mejorando la seguridad de los pacientes: estudio de los incidentes en los cuidados de enfermería Chile [Internet]. 2013. pp. 1-9. Available from: http://www.scielo.br/pdf/reeusp/v47n5/es_0080-6234-reeusp-47-05-1098.pdf [citado 30 de noviembre 2018]

[8] Meléndez M y otros. Percepción del personal de enfermería hacia la cultura de seguridad en un hospital pediátrico en México [Internet]. 2015. Disponible en: https://revistacuidarte.udes.edu.co/index.php/cuidarte/article/view/92 [citado 30 de noviembre 2018]

[9] Poma V. evaluación a la calidad y seguridad en la atención a pacientes del servicio de Medicina interna del hospital Eugenio espejo, Sangolqui [Internet]. 2015. pp. 1-181. Disponible en: https://repositorio.espe.edu.ec/bitstream/21000/12363/1/T-ESPE-049766.pdf [citado 2 de diciembre 2018]

[10] Ministerio de Sanidad Español. Política Social e Igualdad. Estudio IBEAS Prevalencia de efectos adversos en hospitales de Latinoamérica. Madrid. Ministerio de Sanidad: Política Social e Igualdad; 2010

[11] Ministerio de Salud y Protección Social. Seguridad del paciente, Guía de buenas prácticas para la seguridad del paciente. Bogotá, Colombia [Internet]. 2009. Disponible en: https://www.minsalud.gov.co/sites/rid/Lists/BibliotecaDigital/RIDE/DE/CA/Guia-buenas-practicas-seguridad-paciente.pdf [citado 4 de diciembre 2018]

[12] Ministerio de Salud y protección social. Colombia: Seguridad del paciente y la atención segura; 2012. Disponible en: https://www.minsalud.gov.co/sites/rid/Lists/BibliotecaDigital/RIDE/DE/CA/Guia-buenas-practicas-seguridad-paciente.pdf

[13] Ministerio de Salud y protección social. Resolución 1441 de 2013. Disponible en https://www.minsalud.gov.co/sites/rid/Lists/BibliotecaDigital/RIDE/DE/DIJ/resolucion-1441-de-2013.pdf

[14] Ministerio de Salud y protección social. Resolución 2003 de 2014 [Internet]. 2014. Disponible en: https://

www.minsalud.gov.co/Normatividad_Nuevo/Resoluci%C3%B3n%202003%20de%202014.pdf [citado 2 de diciembre 2018]

[15] Barajas ER, González OS, Vera WT, editors. Seguridad del Paciente Hospitalizado. México: Médica Panamericana; 2007

[16] Ministerio de Protección Social. Lineamientos para la implementación de la Política de Seguridad del Paciente. Santiago de Cali [Internet]. 2012. pp. 35-44. Disponible en: http://calisaludable.cali.gov.co/seg_social/2013_Seguridad_Paciente/libro_seguridad_del_paciente.pdf [citado 5 de diciembre 2018]

[17] Agency for Healthcare Research and Quality. Health Care: Medical errors and patient safety. U.S. Departament of Health y Human Service; 2008. Available in: https://www.ahrq.gov/patient-safety/index.html

[18] Ministerio de Protección Social. Lineamientos para la implementación de la Política de Seguridad del Paciente. Santiago de Cali [Internet]. 2015. pp. 35-44. Disponible en: http://calisaludable.cali.gov.co/seg_social/2013_Seguridad_Paciente/libro_seguridad_del_paciente.pdf [citado 5 diciembre 2018]

[19] Vincent C. Patient Safety. London: Churchill-Livingstone; 2006

[20] Giraldo M. Lineamientos para la implementación de la política de seguridad del paciente en la República de Colombia Bogotá. Revista de Medicina: Junta Directiva. 2009;**30**(2). Disponible en: https://encolombia.com/medicina/revistas-medicas/academedicina/va-81/respuestadelministerio/ [citado 10 diciembre 2018]

[21] Taylor S, Vincen C. System Analysis of clinical incidents: The London protocol. Journal of Patient Safety and Risk Management. 2004;(10):211-220. Disponible en: https://doi.org/10.1258/1356262042368255 [citado 13 diciembre 2018]

[22] Ministerio De La Protección Social. Colombia. La seguridad del paciente y la atención segura. 2013. version 2. Disponible en: https://www.minsalud.gov.co/sites/rid/Lists/BibliotecaDigital/RIDE/DE/CA/Guia-buenas-practicas-seguridad-paciente.pdf

[23] Luengas S. Modelo para gestionar la seguridad del paciente en las instituciones de salud. Centro de gestión hospitalaria, VíaSALUD. 2008;**43**:1-5. Disponible en: http://www.cgh.org.co/imagenes/calidadycultura.pdf [citado 18 diciembre 2018]

[24] Luengas S. Seguridad del paciente: un modelo organizacional para el control sistemático de los riesgos en la atención en salud. Documentos de trabajo de la Fundación Corona. Bogotá: Fundación Corona-Centro de Gestión Hospitalaria; 2009. Disponible en: http://www.cgh.org.co [citado 21 diciembre 2018]

[25] Donabedian A. La investigación sobre la calidad de la Atención Médica. Revista Salud de Seguridad Social del Instituto Mexicano de Seguridad Social, México. 1986;**28**:324-327

[26] Martínez A. Gestión sistémica del error: el enfoque del queso suizo en las auditorias. Rev. INNOTEC GESTION. 2013;(4). Disponible en: https://ojs.latu.org.uy/index.php/INNOTEC-Gestion/article/view/164/pdf

[27] Republica de Colombia. Ministerio de Salud. Resolución 741 del 1997. Por la cual se imparte instrucciones sobre seguridad personal de usuarios para Instituciones y demás Prestadores de Servicio de Salud. Diario oficial. no. 741. Bogotá; 1997. https://www.minsalud.gov.co/sites/rid/Lists/BibliotecaDigital/RIDE/DE/DIJ/RESOLUCION-0741-de-1997.pdf

[28] Aranaz J, Aibar C, Vitaller J, Mira J. Gestión Sanitaria—Calidad y Seguridad de los Pacientes. España: Ediciones Diaz de Santos; 2008. p. 389

[29] Reason J. Human Error. New York: Press Syndicate of the University of Cambridge; 1990. p. 258

[30] Giron J. Enfermería y Seguridad del Paciente [Internet]. 2017. Disponible en: http://www.enfermeriayseguridaddelpaciente.com/2017/05/metodologias-de-analisis-de-eventos.html [citado 9 enero 2018]

Section 3

Nursing Enviroments

Chapter 5

Nurse-Patient Conflict: Verification of Structural Model

Mayumi Uno

Abstract

This chapter focuses on the overlooked area of everyday nursing care in which engaging in the depressive feelings between nurses and patients is not recognized as part of nursing care. To comprehend situations that had been overlooked, a conceptual model was constructed by focusing on nurse-patient conflicts and understanding the perception of both nurses and patients based on phenomena. In the established model, it is considered that the so-called "passion" emanating from one's personality, which is beyond techniques of communication and empathic understanding, is involved; this passion is expressed as an "emotional exchange." In an "emotional exchange," one sends "emotional" messages to whom he/she feels safe to express "emotions" and shares similar emotional world by receiving those "emotional" messages as they are. Such an expression has not been reported previously.

Keywords: nurse-patient relationship, conflict, structural model

1. What is a service

A service is characterized by "intangibles," "simultaneity of production and consumption," "equivalent importance of the results and process" and "co-production with customers." The types of services include "core service," which is at the core of a service product, "sub-service," which is associated with the core service, "contingent service," which adapts to the situation, and "potential service element," which is sought out by customers [1]. Subservice, which does not reflect on customer service at hotels and costs at hospitals, tends to be emphasized in service quality evaluation more so than the core service, including the provision of technology that reflects on costs [2]. Quality service is dependent on the subjective and objective evaluation of customers. Customer satisfaction with regard to service is associated with emotion, which impacts evaluation over time [3]. According to Simomura [4], emotion is a central concept in consumption behavior, and satisfaction with a service and customers' emotions cannot be discussed separately. With respect to customer demand and quality, good quality as perceived by a customer is meeting the customer's demand [5], as well as having a certain level of high knowledge, sensitivity, and values to create a better service [6].

2. Services measured using customer expectations and satisfaction

Parasuraman et al.'s [7] SERVQUAL Instrument (a Multiple-item Scale for Measuring Service Quality) is most widely used for measuring a service based on the difference between expectations and satisfaction [8]. This instrument can measure not only customer expectations but also their perception of the quality of service that they received [9]. The perception of quality by service recipients is associated with the morale of the service providers and corporate spirit [10, 11]. We must know and understand the expectations of patients to measure quality of health care. In service marketing research, the relation between expectations for a service and perception of the service received is drawing attention [7, 10, 12–14]. Parasuraman et al. [15] evaluated SERVQUAL Instrument (a Multiple-item Scale for Measuring Service Quality), which they reported in 1985, based on psychological diagnosis. Accordingly, SERVQUAL for patient satisfaction with nursing care, namely, SERVQUAL-N, which is a modified version of SERVQUAL for nursing care, was developed [16]. Consequently, service evaluation based on SERVQUAL has been conducted in Europe, North America, and Asia [17–22]. In SERVQUAL, service quality comprises elements of reliability, responsiveness, assurance, empathy, and tangibles. Meanwhile, Shanaki et al. [23] described the effects of empathy toward service quality using tangibles, responsiveness, trust, accessibility, and service recovery. This shows continuous development in research in various academic fields.

3. Focusing on nurse-patient conflict

A nurse must perceive the feelings and emotions of a patient and respond appropriately so that the latter recognizes that he/she is receiving high quality health care. Nurse-patient conflict arises when a patient's expectations are not met and trust is not established. It is ideal for the conflict to be resolved between a nurse and a patient. Patients have feelings that they are not able to tell nurses about, from which a potential conflict can arise. Patients suffer in situations where they perceive conflict, but they are unable to bring it up with the nurses because of reluctance or resignation. Because a patient's perception affects quality evaluation of nursing care, this study focused on nurse-patient conflict and found meaning in understanding nurses' and patients' perception of phenomena. In the field of nursing care, consideration of patients' emotions and response to their feelings have been considered important. To improve quality of nursing care, nurses are required to go beyond the superficial interaction with patients and respond in a way that is backed by academic significance. Patients' evaluation is indispensable to quality nursing care. There is sufficient need for recognizing the fact that patients carry chaotic feelings, which, in turn, must be comprehended to be able to verbalize, document, conceptualize, and generalize such phenomenon. Therefore, this study is significant in that it academically focused on a phenomenon that has been overlooked thus far.

4. Literature review

4.1 Medical and nursing services and patient satisfaction

In general, various elements, including technical factors, interpersonal factors, cost, and environmental factors, influence patient satisfaction. As such, measuring patient satisfaction in diverse scenes of nursing care is a complex task [24–27]. Patient satisfaction is recognized as an important index for service quality [19, 28, 29]. There is a positive correlation between patient satisfaction regarding nursing care and a patient's perception of service quality [30]. There is also a strong correlation between satisfaction with nursing care and general satisfaction [31]. All nursing care activities are associated with a patient's perception of patient satisfaction [32]. Moreover, values regarding patient satisfaction continue to evolve with time [33]. Oxler [34] focused on patient dissatisfaction and reported that commitment on the part of top leaders and staff was required to set aside time for understanding patient needs, thereby resolving complaints from patients and enhancing satisfaction.

4.2 Development of a measurement scale for patient satisfaction and a conceptual model in nursing care

In a study on patient satisfaction in nursing care, Abdellah and Levine [35] reported on patient satisfaction and occupational satisfaction of nurses. Risser [36] developed the Patient Satisfaction Scale (PSS) for measuring patient satisfaction with primary care nurses and nursing care. Research has advanced, starting with the analysis of the "patient satisfaction" concept regarding modern nursing care [37], incorporation of outpatients' perception into the definition of nursing quality, demonstration of a NEdSERV quality model and development of a scale for service quality in nursing education [38]. These research activities led to the development of a patient-oriented scale for measuring service quality in the outpatient department [39]. In a survey conducted with patients awaiting discharge from the surgical ward of a teaching hospital in Taiwan, a primary care nurse's years of experience as a nurse was found to have affected patient satisfaction [40]. Studies have reported the necessity of an examination focusing on new care models, a partnership care delivery model/core concepts and new models [41], an analysis of patient satisfaction with nursing care using a conceptual nursing framework [33], the development of a satisfaction scale for local nursing care [42], a gap model of care quality in patient-centered nursing care for elucidating concepts of patient-centered care [43], and the development of a scale for measuring satisfaction of critically ill patients [44].

4.3 Nurse-patient relationship

Henderson [45] described her way of understating patients as "getting inside his/her skin," and indicated that nurses should discern the needs of patients before providing nursing care. In the beginning of Interpersonal Aspects of Nursing by Travelbee (1971), Ruth Johnston's (American Journal of Nursing 1971) "Listen, Nurse" was used to emphasize the interpersonal relation that transcends the positions of a nurse and patient. Peplau [46] demonstrated the importance in the encounter between a nurse and a patient and reported that a moral encounter that conveys the understanding of a patient's vulnerability is important. Watson [47] showed that the nurse-patient relationship in nursing science contains intersubjective care and that its practice and process become transpersonal and metaphysical. Reported that a closer relationship is established between a nurse and a patient by shifting the nursing care perspective from organizational goals to patient-centered care (PCC). Cignel [48] considered compassion as an important concept in nurse-patient relationship and argued that compassion as the answer to suffering, which is at the center of care, is equivalent to high-quality care in today's medical care. Described the influence of nurse-patient relationship by stating that the technique used by nurses to draw resources in managing patients, by involving themselves in a patient's phenomenon and distancing themselves, attenuate their suffering that have become involved, but it may keep them from using resources and possibilities gained through interaction with patients. Stated that there is an interrelation within a social relationship, which is characterized by a complementary relationship through self-care based on an existing contractual relationship; Orem said that an ideal relationship would be one in which a patient's and his/her family's stress is reduced and would help them manage matters related to health and health care with a sense of responsibility.

4.4 Trust between nurses and patients

High-quality nursing care is based on trust between nurses and patients. The word "trust" is derived from an old term used to express fidelity and loyalty; this fact has a long history [49]. It is difficult to clearly define nurse-patient trust based on literature [50–52]. Reported that a patient's trust in a nurse is a necessary element for establishing a connection between the patient and that nurse.

Despite the lack of a clear definition of trust, trust affects whether a patient accepts care and treatment [53–55] and is an important factor in a nurse-patient relationship [51, 56]. Johns [57] suggested medical benefits, vulnerability, dependency, and participation in a care plan as being part of a conceptual framework of nurse-patient trust. Meanwhile, Belcher [58] stated that nurses need to act as good communicators to establish a close relationship with a patient while building trust.

4.5 Transition of the concepts of nursing quality until the 2000s and universality

In the 1950s, various nursing theories by nursing theorists were published in countries, including the United States. Starting with "Interpersonal relations in nursing" by Peplau [59] and the "Textbook of the principles and practice of nursing" by Harmer and Henderson [60], Johnson [61] argued that nursing requires care that must be provided by nurses to patients. Subsequently, nursing was considered as being based on interpersonal and personal relationships [62, 63]. As a result, mutual relationship drew attention. After Meyeroff's [64] report on caring was published, caring drew attention in the 1970s. Human caring has been referred as concern and respect for others [65]. Considered caring as the heart and soul of nursing from the viewpoint of the diversity and universality of cultural care. Watson [47] placed nursing in relation to metaphysics and indicated that care is the essence of nursing; she also noted that caring is able to utilize humanity as common sense in intersubjective interaction as defined by phenomenology while suggesting an interrelationship between souls. Based on theorists' conceptual analyses of caring, Morse et al. [66] classified caring into the following five categories: (1) caring as a human state (Lininger et al.), (2) caring as an affect (Babes), (3) caring as a moral imperative or ideal (Watson et al.), (4) caring as an interpersonal relationship (Gardo et al.), and (5) caring as a nursing intervention (Brown et al.). Therefore, in the 1960s and the 1970s, the nomenclature of primary phenomena in nursing science was established because of the clear need for detaching nursing from practice based on medical models [45, 67, 68]; (Rogers, 1970). Nursing concepts in Japan have been affected by claims of theorists who underwent these changes. The theory of human caring became widely known in Japan when Watson visited the country around 1990. Human care, whose main focus is on transpersonal care, has a high affinity with the spiritual culture of the East, and it appears to have been accepted as the essence of universal nursing care.

4.6 Transition of the concepts of nursing quality in recent years and universality

Around 2000, the importance of evidence-based practice (EBP) for high quality nursing was emphasized. It was defined as an important perspective for nurses when taking action as a professional [69–72]. Sackett et al. [71] pointed out that

EBP did not contain the opinions and decision-making of patients along with scientific evidence.

Patient centered care (PCC), along with nurse-patient relationship, was considered the basis for nursing care. PCC drew universal attention as being a form of active nursing intervention including sympathy and empathy [73–75]. Sidani [76] defined PCC as the provision of excellent service and improvement of quality patient care. Meanwhile, the Agency for Healthcare Research and Quality (AHRQ 2001) stated that placing an emphasis on PCC improves the quality of interaction between patients and health care providers and empowers patients in the process. EBP and PCC do not conflict one another and should not be considered separately. Burman [77] emphasized that EBP is among the cornerstones for providing better nursing care to patients. Burman also noted that the integration of EBP and PCC is essential for the health management of patients and the cultivation of organizational culture by nurses and other highly motivated clinicians to provide interdisciplinary PCC is required.

4.7 Empathy

The term empathy was used by Robert Vischer, a German psychologist, in 1873. It was derived from the German word Einfühlung. It was born from the esthetics of the time, which belonged to psychology that considered the empirical/aesthetical/psychological aspects as important [78]. Empathy is the ability to share others' thoughts and emotions [79]. It facilitates proactive behavior toward others and promotes social interaction as well as tolerant relationships. It is cultivated through time-dependent change as a person undergoes the developmental process. This ability appears in early childhood, develops in complex form from school age to adolescence (Eisenberg et al., 2002) [80], and continues from adulthood to old age [81, 82]. Empathy training facilitates the development of emotional abilities in school-age children, promotes skills and friendship [83], and enhances social conduct in adulthood [84]. The concept of empathy includes cognitive empathy, which allows one to sense the emotions of others and enables intentional thinking to a certain extent, and emotional empathy, which is accompanied by physical responses that are difficult to intentionally control [85, 86]. Gutsell and Inzlicht [87] described empathy from three perspectives: behavioral empathy, physical empathy, and subjective empathy.

4.8 Empathy in nursing

Research on empathy has a long history in disciplines, such as psychology and sociology. In nursing science, research has been conducted based on these academic backgrounds. Empathy has been considered as a primary basic concept in nurse-patient relationships and nursing practice. Ens [88] defined empathy as a complex part of the concept of countertransference, whereas Roger [89] argued that countertransference is an inevitable factor in a nurse-patient relationship. Scott [90] maintained that empathy is based on moral perception. Empathy is said to be a technique developed for counseling in the field of psychology [91]. However, Nightingale had used "sympathy" to refer to nurse-patient relationships before the term empathy was used. The reasoning that "nurses must be kind and sympathetic at all times, but they should never be emotional" is based on the recognition that this quality as a nurse assists the treatment process in a nurse-patient relationship [59]. Olso [92] found that there was a correlation between empathy shown by nurses and quality of nursing care. Erikson [93] defined empathy as the ability to show concern for suffering and demonstrated that nurses are required to perceive the suffering of patients so that the latter are able to feel their human dignity being maintained. Erikson [94] stated that nurses must find the desires, trust, hope, powerlessness, guilt, and shame of patients to alleviate the latter's suffering and must understand each patient's unique experience with, knowledge of, and way of feeling toward his/her disease [93, 95]. Hence, empathy can be said to be the basis of therapeutic relationships in nurse-patient relationships.

4.9 What is suffering

Suffering refers to feelings and emotions necessary for those with disease, disability, and life issues to live, which form their experiences. For instance, this includes a diagnosis before birth made possible with medical advances, congenital disorders, chronic diseases, mental illnesses, and situations in which death is impending [63, 96]. According to Frankl [97], who is a psychiatrist heavily influenced by Freud and Adler, suffering is not something that one is born with but rather something one acquires. This is expressed as the "ability to suffer" and some consider that suffering cannot even be acquired if one is emotionless. Travelbee [63] stated that suffering, as with a disease, is an everyday life experience that befalls anyone and defines a status where an individual encounters suffering and experiences suffering at its worst as a malignant phase of despair non-caring and the terminal phase of apathetic indifference. Kato (2004) described suffering from a philosophical/ethical standpoint as primary and secondary suffering. Primary suffering is the anguish/suffering of those that seek help, whereas secondary suffering is suffering caused by a lack of response, inappropriate response, or failure/injustice/malice inherent in the action of responding.

4.10 Patient's suffering and nurse's caring

Travelbee [63] suggested that suffering is accompanied by caring, that vulnerability to suffering is related to the ability range and depth of caring, and that the lack of caring ability induces strong suffering. This means that nurses attempt to truly understand the experiences and feelings unique to a patient [93, 95]. Mayeroff [98] stated that caring practice is formed when those involved share time and place by "being together" and "living together," and emphasized the continuous relationship between the two. Ukigaya [99] indicated that nurses are also cared for by patients and that care has a bi-directional effect. Studies on patients' suffering and nursing care must show that nurses are prepared to identify the suffering of patients for them to feel that their dignity is honored.

Various studies on critical life situations, mental problems, and end-of-life suffering have been conducted. However, no study focuses on patients' emotions (secondary suffering) and shows that nursing (service) is no other than engaging with them.

4.11 Conflict research and its transition

Conflict research has long been conducted in the fields of, among others, psychology and sociology. Robbins [100] defined conflict as a process that starts when one perceives that others have exerted or are attempting to exert a negative effect on matters he/she considers important. No other problems are as strongly connected to emotion as when a conflict arises in interpersonal relationships and emotional changes accompany the occurrence of a conflict. In other words, Robbins stated that conflicts cannot be resolved effectively if one disregards the emotional element of a conflict and attempts to resolve them based on rationality and logic.

4.12 Conflict research in medical care and nursing

Marquis and Huston [101] defined conflict as arising from differences in values, expectations, and backgrounds. They suggested that "cultivation of a mutual relationship and sharing of understanding" are required for patients and medical professionals to maintain a positive relationship. They and stated that conflict arises when the personal relationship is no longer smoothly maintained [102]. Reports on patients' specific situations, difficult patients [103], acute psychiatric wards [104], comparison of home care and nursing homes for older adults [105], and ways to respond to a conflict in specific scenes have been published in clinical conflict research since 2005. Nurses tend to use mutual dialog instead of engaging in a conflict in a stern manner to resolve conflicts in nursing situations [106]. Nurse-patient relationship is fundamental in partnership in nursing and interaction is required to maintain a positive relationship [107].

4.13 Definition of terms

Conflict: In this study, conflict does not refer to evidential conflicts (e.g., medical disputes), but rather to nurse-patient mood discrepancies and emotions.

4.14 Ethical considerations

We explained to all eligible participants that the data obtained in this study would not be used to identify any individuals or used outside of this study; further, it would be strictly managed and destroyed upon completion of the study.

Furthermore, we explained to the nurses that participation was voluntary, refusal to participate would not be disadvantageous to them in any way, participation had no relationship with their course evaluation, and we would consider their submission of the survey form as their having consented to participate.

By contrast, in our explanation to the phone counselors, we assured them that participation in the interview was voluntary, had no relationship with their company performance evaluation, and they could rescind their consent to participate at any time. We obtained permission to use the existing data from the copyright holders.

This study was conducted under the approval of our institution's research ethics committee.

5. Related research history and the position of the present study

As shown in the literature review, when a person makes some kind of value judgment, the emotion associated with the service received rather than the actual service received or the fact that he/she received the service affects the evaluation. Customer response to a service has been researched and systematized in business administration as direct purchasing and consumer choice behaviors. In the medical field, efforts have been made to adapt customer satisfaction and consumer choice behavior, which have been systematized in business administration, to clinical practice.

The focus of the present study is everyday nursing settings in which patients are in a specific (non-critical) situation. A patient suffers when he/she senses that a nurse regards his/her existential value lightly. A patient's anguish/suffering constitutes primary suffering; secondary suffering is caused by a nurse's lack of response to the primary suffering or a nurse's inappropriate response or when failure/injustice/malice is inherent in a nurse's action of responding. In the present study, I focused on nurse-patient conflict to understand patients' suffering and nurses' and patients' perception of suffering. The reason this study focused on conflict is that a conflict is caused by emotional differences resulting from changes in the nurse-patient relationship. There is no study that focuses on the perception of patients, who are the service receivers, and bi-directionally examines the perception of nurses and patients with a focus on the sensing of emotional fluctuations and thoughts. Therefore, in this study, patients' unspoken thoughts were verbalized and a conceptual model for phenomena, which have been overlooked by focusing on nurse-patient conflict in medical treatment settings, was constructed.

6. Conceptual framework of the study

Stages 1–4 of Robbins' [100] framework for the conflict process was applied as follows to nurse-patient conflicts in nursing settings where patients' status was non-critical.

Stage 1 (potential opposition): elements latent in the occurrence of a conflict.

Stage 2 (cognition and personalization): scenes in which a conflict occurs <Recognition>.

Stage 3 (behavior): response (in expectation of problems).

Stage 4 (outcomes): outcomes (of a successfully maintained/built positive relationship).

7. Purpose of the study

The present study focused on areas that have been overlooked in everyday nursing scenes in which engaging with the depressing feelings of patients arising in nurse-patient relationships is not recognized as nursing. To understand the circumstances that have been overlooked, the present study focused on nurse-patient conflict and aimed to understand phenomena from the perspective of both nurses and patients and to establish a conceptual model.

8. Research methods

8.1 Survey participants

1. Nurses

For a descriptive survey on nurses, this study involved 320 nurses that participated in a nursing manager workshop organized by a local nursing professional association in Japan. The reason for the selection was that they had gained appropriate nursing experience as a manager and that their experiences could be verbalized.

2. Telephone counselors (patients' end)

For a survey on patients, because it was difficult to obtain data by interviewing patients directly in line with the intent of the present study, we interviewed eight telephone counselors. Telephone counselors belong to an incorporated non-profit organization whose members comprise non-medical professionals located in Osaka Prefecture, Japan. The organization provides consultations geared toward people for patients with feelings that they were not able to convey to medical professionals.

8.2 Survey process

1. Nurses

In the descriptive survey on nurses, they were instructed to recall nurse-patient conflicts and describe them. Age and years of nursing experience at the time of conflict were recorded as personal characteristics.

2. Telephone counselors (patients)

In the interviews with telephone counselors, they were instructed to recall consultations regarding nurse-patient conflicts. It was confirmed that existing data could be organized in a similar structure to data obtained through the interviews. With regard to personal characteristics, we referred to the age (age range) of patients who called in for a consultation and telephone counseling history of the telephone counselors.

9. Data obtained

In the descriptive survey on nurses, 72 scenes were subjected to analysis after 72 scenes were collected and evaluated to determine whether they were in line with the intent of the present study. In the interviews with telephone counselors, verbatim records of all the interviews were made, and 72 scenes were subjected to analysis.

10. Results

10.1 Gap in perception between nurses and patients

When a conflict arose, systematic thinking, including logical thinking based on EBP and empathic understanding of patients based on PCC, was observed in nurses. Meanwhile, patients carried fragmented emotions, such as "anxiety," "sorrow," "dejection," and "anger." In other words, when I simultaneously looked at the perception of nurses and patients, there was a gap in perception, which was observed as "nurses' systematic understanding" and "patients' fragmented emotions."

10.2 Positive interaction as a result of nurses recognizing the gap in perception

After looking at the perception of nurses and patients simultaneously, we found that there was a gap observed as "nurses' systematic understanding" and "patients' fragmented emotions." When a nurse recognizes this gap in perception, a nurse senses the fragmented emotions that a patient carries while engaging in systematic thinking and understanding. Alternatively, the gap was naturally filled by the nurse placing himself/herself in the patient's shoes to understand the latter's emotions, then a positive interaction would be observed when the nurse expressed empathic understanding toward the patient and shared his/her suffering.

10.3 Suffering based on the gap in perception between nurses and patients and a positive interaction model

In Study 1, we showed that the empathic attitude of a nurse, who recognized the gap between the nurse and patient, resonated with the patient at a soul level. This resulted in a positive interaction where the gap in perception between the nurse and patient was recognized, enabling emotional exchange. Building on these findings,

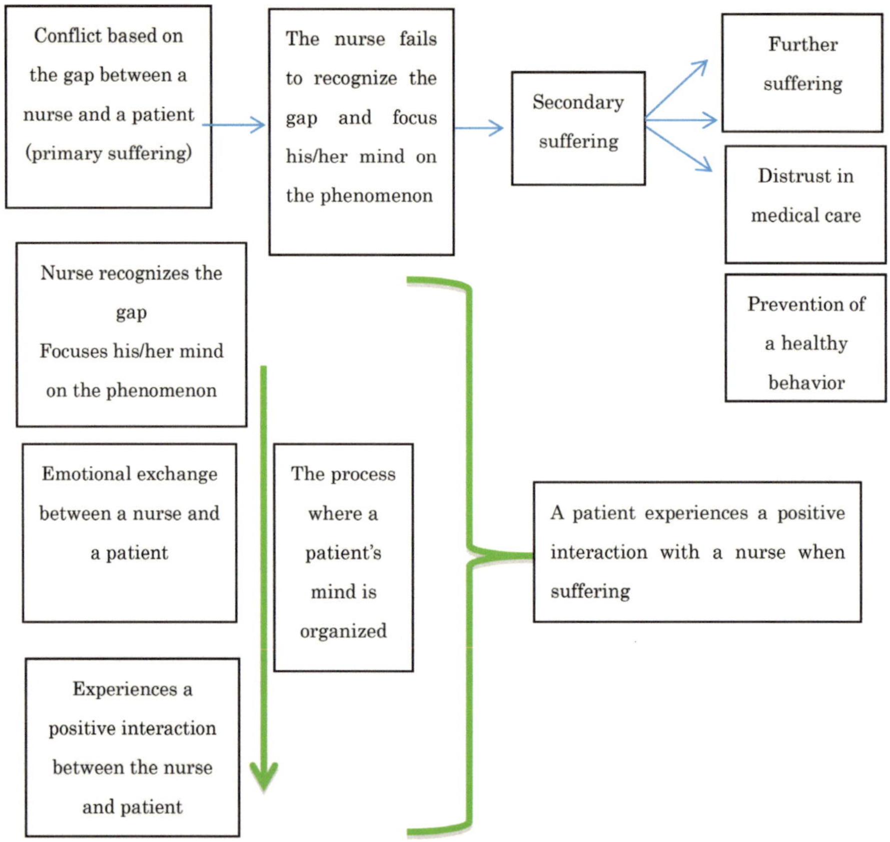

Figure 1.
Suffering based on the gap in perception between a nurse and a patient, and a positive interaction model.

I constructed a model for suffering based on the gap in perception between nurses and patients, and positive interaction (**Figure 1**).

10.4 Structure and definition of the constructed conceptual model

The perception and cognition of phenomena that occur in nursing settings differ between nurses and patients. Nurses encounter various situations related to patients' life and death and experience emotional fluctuations associated with them on a daily basis. Meanwhile, life change caused by hospitalization, although it may be for a short period, is a once, if not only a few times, in a lifetime experience for the patients. As such, because nurses and patients are in different positions, they have different ways of understanding a phenomenon and standards of perception. I elucidated this difference as a gap. Based on what has been described, suffering experienced by a patient was defined as primary suffering. With regard to primary suffering, if the nurse does not recognize conflict and the gap that causes it, the patient will notice the nurse's lack of awareness of it. In other words, the patient experiences secondary suffering when he/she instinctively and intuitively senses the nurse is not truly willing to help the patient who is experiencing primary suffering. As a result, the patient suffers even more, giving rise to distrust in medical care, interfering with his/her health behavior.

If the nurse adequately understands the gap that caused the conflict and comes to feel the emotions of the patient unintentionally and in a natural way, emotional exchange takes place; this cultivates a positive interaction. This process is considered the "process by which the patient's mind is adjusted."

11. Discussion: examination of nurses' and patients' perception of the cause of nurse-patient conflict

11.1 Cause of nurse-patient conflict

Nurses interact with patients at a more intimate level than other health care workers and are committed to life-threatening moments and important life events. As such, nurses have more opportunities to obtain information about patients. Excess and insufficient information can cause conflict. Nurses also witness patients undergoing a great deal of emotional fluctuations. However, they are anxious because they feel that they may no longer be able to engage in "nursing work" if they accept patients' emotions as they are. Washida [108] described such situation as the critical point in clinical practice and where the patients suffer. In several ways, nurses are unable to put it together unless they become objective and distance themselves from emotional fluctuations. It may be that they are able to continue "nursing work" by unconsciously numbing their emotions. The data have shown that conflict is attributable to the gap between nurses and patients.

11.2 Potential opposition of conflict and suffering

The data of the present study was obtained by applying Robbins's [100] framework for conflict process. Nurse-patient communication and trust are believed to be involved in potential opposition. As Usui [109] stated, laypeople remain in a limited understanding of superficial phenomena, whereas experts can penetrate the internal structure of the subject with the help of expert knowledge. Nursing professionals are able to and are expected to enter into a patient's inner state and respond accordingly. However, when nurses are unable to meet these expectations, secondary suffering arises, and patients experience even more anguish.

11.3 Gap in perception between nurses and patients caused by conflict

1. Perception of nurses and patients caused by conflict.

   There was a gap in perception between nurses and patients with regard to conflict. It was observed that nurses tended to understand phenomena using logical thinking, based on EBP, and empathic understanding, based on PCC. This is because nurses were trained as professionals and accustomed to understanding perceived phenomena using scientific thinking and grasping a patient's feelings based on clinical experience. By contrast, patients, who had not received specialized education and whose physical condition had deteriorated, perceived and responded to phenomena with fragmented emotions. Therefore, there was a gap in the perception between nurses and patients. There appears to be a gap between the experience of nurses and patients as humans systematize their experiences and attempt to give them meaning ([89], p. 88).

2. Four aspects of nurse-patient perception gap.

   There was a difference in perception between nurses and patients in situations where a conflict had arisen. There was a gap in communication between them in terms of communication for conveying their perception. In a nurse-patient relationship, communication is not only limited to the process of simply sending/receiving verbal or non-verbal messages but also includes a wider range of information [110]. A gap is created when one fails to receive the information sent. In addition, it has been suggested that communication aimed at ensuring quality of nursing helps develop a positive nurse-patient relationship [111–113]. Attention should also be paid to the relation between the two.

3. Nurses' recognition of the perception gap.

There was a gap in perception between nurses and patients in situations where a conflict had arisen. Whether nurses recognize this gap affects the way they influence patients. Nurses will not give any thought to patients' emotions unless they are aware of the gap. Recognizing the gap between nurses and patients is the first step in achieving true empathy.

11.4 Emotional exchange between nurses and patients

11.4.1 Emotional exchange

In the present study, we also focused on the fact that patients come to experience an emotion because of conflict. Emotional exchange was defined as sending "emotional" messages to whom one feels safe to express "emotions" and share his/her emotional world as a result of them receiving those "emotional" messages as they are.

Nurses were able to notice and share patients' anguish owing to the empathic interaction in which they recognized the gap with patients. Emotional intelligence (EI), which is the ability to sense patients' emotions, on the nurses' part is believed to be involved in the process. EI is the ability to understand emotion accurately, utilize emotion to facilitate recognition, and reflect on emotion [114], in addition to one's own motivation and human relationship skills (Goleman 1995). EI was internationally acknowledged as a result of Goleman's (1998) "Working with Emotional Intelligence." Nurses, whose profession involves interaction with others, are required to have a high level of EI, particularly the ability to sense patients' emotions and respond accordingly.

11.4.2 Empathy and suffering

The word empathy was derived from the Greek word "empatheia," which was formed by combining em (to attempt to insert) and patheia (suffering). The Oxford English Dictionary defines empathy as "the ability to project personality on the subject of reflection (and to perfectly understand it)." It is a term primarily related to the field of psychology.

We believe that feeling a patient's feelings/intentions and standing by them are equal to showing an interest in his/her concerns. Nurses are equipped with not only the ability to logically understand matters but also the sensitivity to acknowledge the emotions patients experience as a person. Intentional empathy is often considered as the act of entering into others' emotions [115]. To stand by the patients, it is key to interact with them while acknowledging the gap and for nurses to place themselves in the thoughts of patients.

11.4.3 Sharing of suffering

Patients are in a state of distress, and they find the act of conveying the fact painful (suffering). Moreover, they suffer from the pain of not being empathized and understood. In short, their suffering is two-fold. Emotions of "anxiety," "sorrow," "dejection," and "anger" experienced by patients constitute primary suffering;

secondary suffering arises when they are unable to engage in emotional exchange with nurses [99]. Even if patients' suffering is not resolved altogether when a conflict arises, showing concern for their suffering and approaching their wishes by coming from the same state are considered sharing of suffering. Nurses must show concern to patients' emotions, which Nightingale [116] called the question about "the understanding of the things one is in the process of doing"; it is "the ability to put oneself in another person's shoes, the ability to understand intuitively what that person needs, and the ability to take on the fate of that person." These are unique to nursing.

12. Examination of the suffering based on the perception of nurses and patients, and the significance and validity of a good interaction model

In the present study, we focused on the mentally/physically non-critical situations of patients in which issues, such as patients' depressive feelings that do not pose a medical or nursing problem, were not recognized as requiring nursing intervention and thus overlooked. The purpose of the study was to elucidate this concept.

Data showed that both experienced and newly recruited nurses with an active imagination had an intuition that "something was different about the patients," or "something had happened," or "something was wrong." An "awakening" takes place when one intuitively grasps a patient and distances oneself from this understanding. How, then, is this possible? This is achieved by providing nursing care while caring for a patient and wishing to understand the inner state of that person, that is, "passion" exuding from a nurse's personality that is beyond the technical limits of communication skills and empathic understanding. It may be technically possible for a nurse to perceive a gap and attempt to focus his/her mind on phenomena. However, to go a step further, techniques alone are not enough. Patients must be able to feel that they are fortunate to have met the nurse and are emotionally relieved. We were able to demonstrate that striving to be such a nurse results in high-quality nursing practice and shows the profundity of a practice involving humans.

"Passion" exuding from nurses is said to fall under the scope of nurses' individual ability. This area has been regarded as part of personal capability and appeal. It has not been academically studied because of the lack of clear training methods or evaluation indices for exploring it. However, without considering the relationship with patients and giving thought to this area, true improvement of quality as perceivable by patients is not possible. I was able to suggest the need for academic inquiry by the model of the present study.

13. Validity examination of the conceptual model by clinicians and its contribution to clinical practice

We explained the purpose/results of the present study and the final model to clinicians to ask for their opinions and examine the validity of the model. We asked for the opinions of three individuals with 30–40 years of nursing experience, who understood the intent of the present study, and who previously worked in acute wards and currently belong to the field of visiting nursing care.

First, it should come as no surprise that the relationship with patients does not deepen by examining the horizontal line (the flow from primary to secondary suffering) of the model. In fact, we visited patients who experienced secondary suffering as visiting nurses. Therefore, it was approved that nurses' involvement with primary suffering was important based on the opinion that "a patient may not have been so stubborn if the nurses had engaged at a slightly deeper level during the hospitalization period." Next, based on the examination of the vertical line (the flow from primary suffering to positive interaction), it was agreed upon that in some cases, a positive encounter with a nurse may be more important than curing the disease itself. In recent years, being able to engage in emotional exchange with nurses provides a positive interaction experience for those who are more than likely to have no one close-by to understand them, as an extremely large number of patients are living with chronic diseases and family morphology changes as they age. Consequently, clinicians endorsed the validity of the model. It was shown that there is a need to recognize this study's model in and its possible contribution to clinical practice. Therefore, I believe that the model created in this study represents everyday scenes for nurses and patients and is useful for reaffirming the fact that it was overlooked and not recognized.

14. Conclusion

Nurse-patient relationship as a result of nurse-patient conflict depends on the way one looks at "communication" and "trust." Its interaction may involve drawing strength from patients as the power of nursing. It was shown that sharing of suffering by emotional exchange was a key concept for it. Washida [108] stated that the relationship between those being admitted and those accepting them is reversed in hospitals. Washida added that clinical settings are the critical plane on which those receiving care and those providing care come in contact in an inverted manner. The nurses working there become partly exhausted because of work responsibilities and the physical demands of work, but more so because they experience extreme emotional fluctuations multiple times a day. These emotional fluctuations rarely happen to average people. Amid these fluctuations, nurses are believed to maintain their balance by unconsciously getting out of touch with patients' myriad emotions and feelings while using scientific thinking at all times to avoid being affected by these fluctuations. With regard to the difficulty in listening, Kawai et al. (2003, p. 211) stated that "narrative does not trickle down in front of those who look for narrative, while it reveals itself only a little to those who patiently wait for it." Kawai and colleagues explained: "unless one is convinced that others will accept whatever he/she says and that they will follow through with the various problems that may arise as a result of him/her speaking out, he/she will not speak about the entangled thoughts he/she has. To speak means one becomes multiplexed in front of others and will unstably float around with no visible landing point." Patients suffering from a disease have a heightened sensitivity. They are probably able to intuitively sense whether nurses that are taking care of them are mature on the inside. What is important to patients is that nurses make an earnest effort to engage with them. They are pleased with this effort, and they perhaps do not expect nurses to completely understand them, the patients who are in great distress.

Acknowledgements

Partial additions and modifications were made to my dissertation for the doctoral program at Osaka University Graduate School in the present study.

Author details

Mayumi Uno
Faculty of Nursing, Shijonawate-Gakuen University, Osaka, Japan

*Address all correspondence to: unomayu@gmail.com

References

[1] Kondo T. Service Marketing: Service Product Development and Customer Value Creation. 2nd ed. Seisansei Shuppan; 2010

[2] Lages LF, Fernandes JC. The SERVQUAL scale: A multi-item instrument for measuring service personal values. Journal of Business Research. 2005;**58**:1562-1572

[3] Iacobucci D, Grayson KA, Ostorm AL. The calculus of service quality and customer satisfaction. Advances in Services Marketing and Management. 1994;**3**:9-15

[4] Simomura B. Achievement as gift and prestige: Formulating anticipated emotion of others as new determinant of consumer motivation. ASEAN Marketing Journal. 2016;**8**(1):29-53

[5] Uehara N, Kuroda S, Iizuka Y, et al. Medical Quality Management System: The Use of ISO 9001 in Medical Institutions. Tokyo: Japanese Standards Association; 2003

[6] Takano N. The Moment Valued by Ritz Carlton where Service Is Surpassed. Tokyo: Kanki Shuppan; 2013

[7] Parasuraman A, Zeithaml V, Berry L. A conceptual model of service quality and its implications for future research. Journal of Marketing. 1985;**49-Fall**:41-50

[8] Korner MM. The conceptual domain of service quality for inpatients nursing services. Journal of Business Research. 2000;**48**:267-283

[9] Randy WC, Leigh AC. Measuring functional service quality using SERVQUAL in a high-dependence health service relationship. The Health Care Manager. 2007;**26**(4):306-317

[10] Parasuraman A, Zeithaml V, Berry L. A multiple-item scale for measuring consumer perceptions of service quality. Journal of Retailing. 1988;**64**(1):12-40

[11] Parasuraman A, Berry L, Zeithmal V. Refinement and reassessment of the SERVQUAL scale. Journal of Retailing. 1991;**67**(4):420-447

[12] Carman JM. Consumer perceptions of service quality: An assessment of the SERVQUAL dimensions. Journal of Retailing. 1990;**66**(1):33-55

[13] Finn DW, Lamb CW Jr. An evaluation of the SERVQUAL scale in a retailing setting. Advanced Consumer Research. 1991;**18**(1):483-490

[14] Zeithaml VA, Parasuraman A, Berry LL. Problems and strategies in service marketing. Journal of Marketing. 1988;**49**(2):33-48

[15] Parasuraman A, Berry L, Zeithmal V. Alternative scale for measuring service quality: A comparative assessment based on psychometric and diagnostic criteria. Journal of Retailing. 1994;**70**(3):201-230

[16] Scardina SA. SERVQUAL: A tool for evaluating patient satisfaction with nursing care. Journal of Nursing Care Quality. 1994;**8**(2):38-46

[17] Chou SM, Chen TF, Woodard B. Using SERVQUAL to evaluate quality disconfirmation of nursing service in Taiwan. Journal of Nursing Research. 2005;**13**(2):75-84

[18] Curry A, Stark S. Quality of service in nursing homes. Health Service Management Research. 2000;**13**(4):205-215

[19] Gonzalez-Valentin A, Padin-Lopez S, Ramon-Garrido E. Patient satisfaction with nursing care regional university

hospital in southern Spain. Journal of Nursing Care Quality. 2005;**20**(1):63-72

[20] Lee MA, Yom YH. A comparative study of patient's and nurses' perceptions of the quality of nursing service. International Journal of Nursing Study. 2007;**44**(4):543-555

[21] Lumby J, England K. Patient satisfaction with nursing care in colorectal surgical population. International Journal of Nursing Practice. 2000;**6**(3):140-145

[22] Uzun O. Patient satisfaction with nursing care at a university hospital in Turkey. Journal of Nursing Care Quality. 2001;**8**(2):38-46

[23] Shanaki M, Ranjbar V, Shakhsian F. Investigation on relationship between service quality and customer satisfaction (case study in Iranian Shahid Rajayi port). Indian Journal of Science and Technology. 2012;**5**(12):111-120

[24] Avis M, Bond M. Satisfying solutions: A review of some unresolved issues in the measurement of patient satisfaction. Journal of Advanced Nursing. 1995;**22**:316-322

[25] Chang K. Dimensions and indicators of patients' perceived nursing care quality in the hospital setting. Journal of Nursing Care Quality. 1977;**11**:26-37

[26] O'Connell B, Young J, Twigg D. Patient satisfaction with nursing care: A measurement conundrum. International Journal of Nursing Practice. 1999;**5**:72-77

[27] Zahr LK, William SG, El-Hadad A. Patient satisfaction with nursing care in Alexandria, Egypt. Journal of Nursing Studies. 1991;**28**:337-342

[28] Currie V, Harvey G, West E, Mckenna H, Kenney S. Relationship between quality of care, staffing levels, skill mix and nurse autonomy: Literature review. Journal of Advanced Nursing. 2005;**1**:73-82

[29] Sahin B, Yilmaz F, Lee KH. Factors affecting inpatient satisfaction: Structural equation modeling. Journal of Medical System. 2007;**31**:9-16

[30] Neidz BA. Correlates of hospitalized patients' perceptions of service quality. Research in Nursing & Health. 1988;**21**:339-349

[31] Beck KL, Larrabee JH. Measuring patients' perception of nursing care. Nursing Management. 1996;**27**:32-34

[32] Oflaz F, Vural H. The evaluation of nurses and nursing activities through the perceptions of inpatients. International Nursing Review. 2010;**57**(2):232-239

[33] Wagner D, Bear M. Patient satisfaction with nursing care: A concept analysis within a nursing framework. Journal of Advanced Nursing. 2009;**65**(3):692-701

[34] Oxler KF. Achieving patient satisfaction: Resolving patient complaints. Holistic Nursing Practice. 1997;**11**(4):27-34

[35] Abdellah FG, Levine E. Developing a measure of patient and personnel satisfaction with nursing care. Nursing Research. 1957;**5**(3):100-108

[36] Risser NL. Development of an instrument to measure patient satisfaction with nurses and nursing care in primary care setting. Nursing Research. 1975;**24**(1):45-52

[37] Mahon PY. An analysis of the concept 'patient satisfaction' as it relates to contemporary nursing care. Nursing Standard. 1996;**10**:34-38

[38] Roberts P. The development of NEdSERV: Quantitative

instrumentation to measure service quality in nurse education. Nurse Education Today. 1999;**19**:396-407

[39] Hiidenhovi H, Laippala P, Nojonen K. Development of a patient-oriented instrument to measure service quality in outpatient departments. Journal of Advanced Nursing. 2001;**34**(5):696-705

[40] Chin HH. Measuring patient satisfaction as an outcome of nursing care at a teaching hospital of Southern Taiwan. Journal of Nursing Care Quality. 2003;**18**(2):143-150

[41] Splaine WM. The partnership care delivery model: An examination of the core concept and the need for a new model of care. Journal of Nursing Management. 2008;**16**:629-638

[42] Cheng LS. Satisfaction scale for community nursing: Development and validation. Journal of Advanced Nursing. 2010;**66**(10):2331-2340

[43] Dabney BW. Service quality and patient-central care. Academy of Medical-Surgical Nurses. 2013;**22**(6):359-364

[44] De-La-Cueva L et al. Development of an instrument to measure the degree of critical patient's satisfaction with nursing care: Research protocol. Journal of Advanced Nursing. 2014;**70**(1):201-210

[45] Henderson AV. The nature of nursing. American Journal of Nursing. 1964;**64**:62-68

[46] Peplau HE. Peplau's theory of interpersonal relations. Nursing Science Quality. 1997;**10**:162-167

[47] Watson. Nursing: Human Science and Human Care. Igaku Shoin; 1998. Translated by Inaoka F et al.

[48] Cignel MVD. Compassion in care: A qualitative study of older people with a chronic disease and nurses. Nursing Ethics. 2011;**18**(5):672-685

[49] Mollering G, Bachmann R, Hee LS. Understanding organizational trust: Foundations, constellations, and issues of operationalisation. Journal of Managerial Psychology. 2004;**19**:556-570

[50] Doucet TJ. Trusting another: A parse research method study. Nursing Science Quarterly. 2009;**22**:259-266

[51] Pask EJ. Trust: An essential component of nursing practice—Implications for nurse education. Nurse Education Today. 1995;**15**(3):190-195

[52] Ramo H. Moments of trust: Temporal and spatial factors of trust in organisations. Journal of Managerial Psychology. 2004;**19**:760-775

[53] Hams SP. Concept analysis of trust: A coronary care perspective. Intensive and Critical Care Nursing. 1997;**13**(6):351-356

[54] Hupcey JE, Penrod J, Moorse JM. An exploration and advancement of the concept of trust. Journal of Advanced Nursing. 2001;**36**(2):282-293

[55] Semmes C. Developing trust: Patient practitioner encounters in natural health care. Journal of Contemporary Ethnography. 1991;**19**(4):450-470

[56] Wallston KA, Wallston BS, Gore S. Development of a scale to measure nurses' trust in patients. Nurse Researcher. 1973;**2**:232-235

[57] Johns JL. A concept analysis of trust. Journal of Advanced Nursing. 1996;**24**:76-83

[58] Belcher M. Graduate nurses' experiences of developing trust in the nurse-patient relationship. Contemporary Nurse. 2009;**31**:142-152

[59] Peplau HE. Interpersonal Relations in Nursing. New York: G.P. Putnam's Sons; 1952; Translated by Inada Y et al.

(1973). Interpersonal Relations in Nursing, Igaku-Shoin

[60] Harmer B, Henderson V. Textbook of the Principles and Practice of Nursing. New York: Macmillan; 1955

[61] Johnson DE. The Nature of Science of Nursing. The Essence of Nursing. Gendaisha; 1959. Translated by Sotoguchi T (1974)

[62] Orlando IJ. The Dynamic Nurse Patient Relationship. New York: G. P. Putnam; 1961

[63] Travelbee J. Interpersonal Aspects of Nursing. Igaku Shoin; 1974. Translated by Hasegawa H et al.

[64] Mayeroff M. On caring. The International Philosophical Quarterly. 1965:462-474

[65] Sobel DE. Human caring. American Journal of Nursing. 1969;**69**(12):2612

[66] Morse JM, Solberg SM, Neaner WL, et al. Comparative analysis of conceptualizations and theories of caring. Advanced in Nursing Science. 1990;**13**(1):1-10

[67] Abdellah FG. The nature of nursing science. Nursing Research. 1969;**18**(5):390-393

[68] Hall LE. Nursing: What is it? The Canadian Nurse. 1964;**60**(2):150-154

[69] French P. What is the evidence on evidence-based nursing? An epistemological concern. Journal of Advanced Nursing. 2002;**37**(3):250-257

[70] Roberts K. Evidence-based practice: An idea whose time has come. Collegian. 1998;**5**(3):24-27

[71] Sackett DL, Rosenberg WMC, Gray JAM, Haynes RB, Richardson WS. Evidence-based medicine: What it is and what it isn't. British Medical Journal. 1996;**312**:71-72

[72] Swan B, Lang N, McGinley A. Perspectives in ambulatory care. Access to quality health care: Links between evidence, nursing language, and informatics. Nursing Economy. 2004;**22**(6):325-332

[73] Canning D, Rosenberg JP, Yates P. Therapeutic relationship in specialist palliative care nursing practice. International Journal of Palliative Nursing. 2007;**13**:222-229

[74] Grandos GG. The nurse–patient relationship as a caring relationship. Nursing Science Quality. 2009;**22**:126-127

[75] Welch M. Pivotal moments in the therapeutic relationship. International Journal of Mental Health Nursing. 2005;**14**:161-165

[76] Sidani S. Effects of patient-centered care on patient outcomes: An evaluation. Research and Theory for Nursing Practice. 2008;**22**:24-37

[77] Burman ME, Robinson B, Hart AM. Linking evidence-based nursing practice and patient-centered care through patient preferences. Nursing Administration Quarterly. 2013;**37**(3):231-241

[78] Depew D. Empathy, psychology, and aesthetics: Reflections on a repair concept. An Interdisciplinary Journal of Rhetorical Analysis and Invention. 2005;**4**(1):99-107

[79] Eisenberg N, Fabes RA. Empathy: Conceptualization, measurement, and relation to prosocial behavior. Motivation and Emotion. 1990;**14**:131-149

[80] Konrath S, O'Brien E, Hsing C. Changes in dispositional empathy in American college students over time: A

meta-analysis. Personality and Social Psychology Review. 2011;**15**:180-198

[81] Grühn D, Rebucal C, Diehl M, Lumley M, Labouvie VG. Empathy across the adult lifespan: Longitudinal and experience-sampling findings. Emotion. 2008;**8**:753-765

[82] O'Brien E, Konarath SH, Grühn D, Hagen AL. Empathic concern and perspective talking: Linear and quadratic effects of age across the adult life span. Journal of Gerontology, Series B: Psychological Sciences and Social Sciences. 2013;**68**:168-175

[83] Greenberg MT, Kusche CA, Cook ET, Quamma JP. Promoting emotional competence in school-aged children: The effects of the PATHS curriculum. Development and Psychopathology. 1995;**7**:117-136

[84] Gibbs JC, Potter GB, Barriga AQ, Liau AK. Developing the helping skills and prosocial motivation of aggressive adolescents in peer group programs. Aggression and Violent Behavior. 1996;**1**:283-305

[85] Deccety J, Lamm C. Human empathy through the lens of social neuroscience. Scientific World Journal. 2006;**6**:1146-1163

[86] Preston SD, Waal FB. Empathy: Its ultimate and proximate bases. Behavioral and Brain Sciences. 2002;**25**:1-20

[87] Gutsell JN, Inzlicht M. Intergroup differences in the sharing of emotive states: Neural evidence of an empathy gap. Social Cognitive and Affective Neuroscience. 2012;**7**:596-603

[88] Ens IC. An analysis of the concept of countertransference. Archives of Psychiatric Nursing. 1988;**7**(5):273-281

[89] Roger BL. Concepts, analysis and the development of nursing knowledge: The evolutionary cycle. Journal of Advanced Nursing. 1989;**14**:330-335

[90] Scott PA. Emotion, moral perception, and nursing practice. Nursing Philosophy. 2000;**1**:123-133

[91] Rogers CR. The necessary and sufficient conditions of therapeutic personality change. Journal of Consulting Psychology. 1957;**21**:91-103

[92] Olso JK. Relationships between nurse-expressed empathy, patient-perceived empathy and patient distress, image. Journal of Nurse Scholarship. 1995;**27**(4):317-322

[93] Eriksson K. Understanding the world of the patient, the suffering human being: The new clinical paradigm from nursing to caring. Advanced Practice Nursing Quarterly. 1997;**3**:8-13

[94] Erikson K. Caring, spirituality and suffering. In: Roach MS, editor. Caring from the Heart: The Convergence of Caring and Spirituality. Mahwah, NJ: Paulist Press; 1997. p. 81

[95] Beech P, Norman IJ. Patients' perception of the quality of psychiatric nursing care: Findings from a small-scale descriptive study. Journal of Clinical Nursing. 1995;**4**:117-123

[96] Kleinman A, Kleinman J. Suffering and its professional transformation: Toward an ethnography of interpersonal experience. In: Kleinmen A, editor. Writing at the Margin: Discourse between Anthropology and Medicine. University of California Press; 1995. pp. 95-119

[97] Frankle VE, Yamada K. Suffering Humans. Tokyo: Shunjusha; 2004. translated by Matsuda M

[98] Mayoroff. The essence of care. In: The Meaning of Life. Yumiru Shuppan; 1987. Translated by Tamura S et al

[99] Ukigaya S. The Hope of Suffering, Anthropology of Suffering by an Expert. Kyodo Isho: Shuppan; 2014

[100] Robbins SP. Organizational Behavior. 8th ed. Japan: Diamond; 2009 [in Japanese]

[101] Marquis BL, Huston CJ. Conflict management. In: Leadership Roles and Management Function in Nursing: Theory and Application. 6th ed. Philadelphia: Wolters Kluwer Health/ Lippincott Williams and Wilkins; 2009

[102] Bissell P, May CR, Noyce PR. From compliance to concordance: Barriers to accomplishing a re-framed model of health care interactions. Social Science & Medicine. 2004;**58**(4):851-862

[103] Baum N. Dealing with difficult patients. Journal of Medical Practice Management. 2009;**July/August**:33-36

[104] Bowers L, Flood C, Brennan G, Allan T. A replication study of the city nurse intervention: Reducing conflict and containment on three acute psychiatric wards. Journal of Psychiatric and Mental Health Nursing. 2008;**15**:737-742

[105] Small JA, Montoro-Rodriguez J. Conflict resolution styles: A comparison of assisted living and nursing home facilities. Journal of Gerontological Nursing. 2006:39-45

[106] Mahon MM, Nicotera AM. Nursing and conflict communication: Avoidance as preferred strategy. Nursing Administration Quarterly. 2011;**35**:152-163

[107] McQueen A. Nurse–patient relationships and partnership in hospital care. Journal of Clinical Nursing. 2000;**9**:723-731

[108] Washida K. The Power of "Listening": An Essay on Clinical Philosophy. Hankyu Communications; 2010

[109] Usui H. Kagakuteki Kangoron. 3rd ed. Nihonkangokyokaisupankai; 1999 [in Japanese]

[110] Sheppard M. Client satisfaction, extended intervention and interpersonal skills in community mental health. Journal of Advanced Nursing. 1993;**18**:246-259

[111] Fosbinder D. Patient perceptions of nursing care: An emerging theory of interpersonal competence. Journal of Advanced Nursing. 1994;**20**:1085-1093

[112] Severston BM. Therapeutic communication demystified. Journal of Nursing Education. 1990;**29**:190-192

[113] Thorsteinsson LSCH. The quality of nursing care as perceived by individuals with chronic illnesses: The magical touch of nursing. Journal of Clinical Nursing. 2002;**11**:32-44

[114] Salovey P, Mayer JD. Emotional Intelligence. Baywood Publishing Co., Inc.; 1990

[115] Golis CC. Empathy Selling. Melbourne: Lothian; 1991

[116] Nightingale F. Notcs on Nursing, What it Is, and What it Is Not, D Appleton and Company; 1860. http://digital.library.upenn.edu/women/nightingale/nursing/nursing.html

Chapter 6

Nursing Environments: Nurses Perspectives

Natasha Khamisa

Abstract

Nurses have been found to experience higher burnout levels compared with other health professionals owing to the nature of their work. High burnout levels among nurses have been attributed to their stressful working environments. Prolonged exposure to work-related stress leading to burnout has negative consequences for job satisfaction and general health of nurses. This has wider implications on the health system, such as high turnover rates and compromised patient care. There is a significant gap in research focusing on the relationship between work-related stress, burnout, job satisfaction and general health of nurses in developing countries such as South Africa. A study exploring the relationships between work-related stress, burnout, job satisfaction and general health among South African nurses over time was conducted in order to inform how best to improve nursing environments while enabling quality nursing practice and patient care. A total of 895 nurses participated in the study at baseline and 277 of these individuals were followed up with a year later. Findings showed that although stress related to security risks in the workplace predicts job satisfaction as well as general health, stress related to patient care and nursing shortages better predict job satisfaction and general health over time. Burnout better predicts job satisfaction than general health over time.

Keywords: work-related stress, burnout, job satisfaction, general health, nurses, South Africa

1. Introduction

The health service industry is increasingly becoming more globalized and liberalized, thereby resulting in a higher demand for skilled health workers. Interdependency and interconnectedness among global societies has led to increased mobility among skilled health workers, resulting in a shortage of health professionals in the health care systems of some countries. South Africa in particular has recently been affected by this trend in international migration of professional nurses, migration of nurses from rural to urban areas as well as migration of nurses from the public sector to the private sector [1]. According to the South African Nursing Council (SANC) the nurse to population ratio is recorded at 197:1 [2].

Given South Africa's nurse driven health system, a shortage of nurses (the gap between supply and demand of 18,758 nurses) makes managing the country's quadruple burden of disease (HIV/AIDS, TB, infectious diseases and under nutrition) challenging [1]. Nurses are forced to adapt to as well as cope with shortages by learning new skills, expanding their capabilities and assuming additional responsibilities, among other coping mechanisms. Such adaptation and adjustment contribute to work-related stress, thereby leading to high levels of burnout, low job satisfaction as well as poor physical and mental wellbeing [3].

Difficult working environments pose serious challenges for patient care and safety while favorable working environments are associated with better job satisfaction, decreased burnout and improved wellbeing of nurses [4]. Healthy working conditions have been shown to improve nurse wellbeing and patient outcomes in developed countries. Several studies conducted in developing countries show that favorable working environments improve staffing levels, thereby improving nurse and patient outcomes [5].

Burnout, defined as long term exhaustion and reduced interest in work [6], is a global phenomenon and has been found to be prevalent among employees whose work is constantly demanding and requires intense interactions of a physical and emotional nature [7]. It is believed that burnout is a manifestation of disconnection between employees and their working environment, whereby primary areas of work life such as reward, control and workload are compromised [8]. Prolonged exposure to these stressors leads to feelings of depersonalisation, whereby nurses lose compassion and sensitivity toward their patients. Depersonalisation negatively affects their ability to evaluate their work in a positive way, resulting in feelings of incompetence and low personal accomplishment. Emotional exhaustion sets in, which makes these nurses feel as if they do not have the emotional energy or resources to cope with the situation [9].

Highest levels of burnout are reported for South African nurses compared to nurses working in other low and middle income countries [10]. This is exacerbated by difficult working conditions characterized by high patient loads, a shortage of staff, increasing job demands and the quadruple burden of disease. Following factor analysis of various stress factors reported by South African nurses, researchers identified five specific stressors that contribute to burnout, namely patient care, staff issues, job demands, lack of support and overtime [11].

Work-related stress is a result of exposure to stressors within working environments that lead to burnout through the depletion of physical and mental resources needed for coping, which is determined by employees' perceptions as well as their emotional responses to levels of threat experienced [12]. Negative perception and appraisal of one's working environment affects job satisfaction [13]. Imbalance between stressful demands of the workplace and resources needed to cope with them affects physical and mental health outcomes (referred to as general health in this manuscript) [14].

Following depletion of physical and mental resources, one's ability to successfully perform tasks and achieve goals is compromised, which explains the association between burnout and job satisfaction. This leads to strain which manifests in the form of poor health outcomes, including headaches, insomnia and depression [3].

For the purpose of this study, the factors identified by Rothmann et al. [11] were referred to as work-related stressors and used to determine the extent to which each one contributes to burnout, job satisfaction and general health of nurses over time. A systematic review of existing literature revealed the following model illustrating relationships between contributing factors and health outcomes of burnout among nurses (**Figure 1**) [15].

Although studies have confirmed that both job satisfaction and burnout are effects of exposure to stressful working environments leading to health consequences [16], the causal nature and direction of these relationships remain

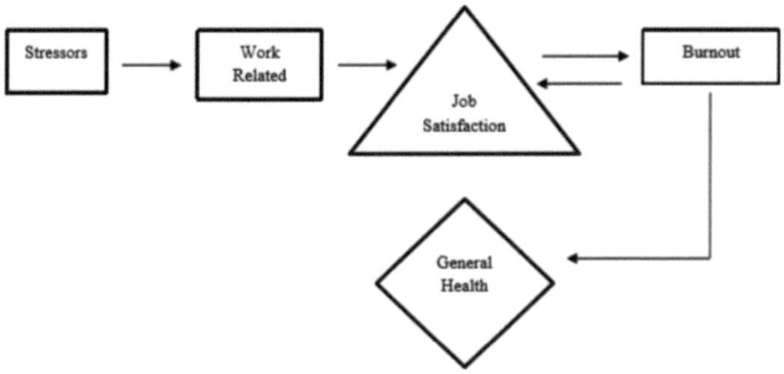

Figure 1.
Existing model illustrating relationships between contributing factors and health outcomes of burnout among nurses.

ambiguous, especially within developing contexts such as South Africa. This study aimed to identify the relationships between work-related stress, burnout, job satisfaction and general health of South African nurses in order to better understand these relationships thereby enabling improvement of working environments and patient care.

2. Methodology

2.1 Participants

Of 1200 invited nurses 895 participated in the baseline study (response rate = 75%). Of these, 277 nurses were followed up a year later. Participants were recruited from two public and two private hospitals using stratified random sampling. Demographic differences were noted between baseline and follow up whereby significant differences were found for age, experience and hours worked per week [17].

2.2 Measurement tools

All participants received five questionnaires to complete. The Socio Demographic Questionnaire consisted of questions pertaining to the age, gender, level of education, level of experience, population group and number of days/hours worked per week. The Nursing Stress Indicator was designed to specifically measure the frequency and severity of five specific stressors identified among South African nurses (patient care, staff issues, supervision/management issues, overtime and job demands). The Maslach Burnout Inventory –Human Services Survey was designed to measure burnout using three sub scales (emotional exhaustion, depersonalization and lack of personal accomplishment) among individuals working in the human services and health care occupations including nursing. The Job Satisfaction Survey measures job satisfaction on nine facets (pay, promotion, supervision, fringe benefits, operating conditions, contingent rewards, co-workers, nature of work and communication) within organisations in the social sector of employment. The General Health Questionnaire was used to detect psychiatric illness as well as current psychological states and perceived quality of life using four sub scales (somatic symptoms, anxiety and insomnia, social dysfunction and severe depression). All questionnaires were reliable and valid within the South African context [17].

2.3 Data collection

Unit managers distributed invitation packs containing an explanatory statement, consent form, five questionnaires and a sealable envelope. Participants returned completed questionnaires and consent forms (including contact details for follow up 1 year later) in sealed envelopes which they placed in sealed boxes. This was accessed by the researcher to ensure privacy and confidentiality of responses. Participants consenting to follow up were contacted to arrange data collection a year later. Participants returned completed follow up questionnaires in a sealed envelope placed in sealed boxes situated around the hospital. These were stored together with respective questionnaires completed at baseline for each participant. Participants were given 3 weeks to complete the questionnaires at both time points with reminders being issued 2 weeks after initial questionnaire distribution [17].

2.4 Design and analysis

The study design used was a longitudinal design. This design involves the collection of data from the same sample over time enabling the observation of changes in outcomes. Longitudinal designs are used to quantify trends, describe progression of events, identify patterns of change and test theory. For these reasons, this design was chosen to examine the relationship between work-related stress, burnout, job satisfaction and general health of nurses over time. This design is suitable because it enables the study of development and natural occurrence of events over time [17].

Data was entered into a statistical package (SPSS version 20) and analyzed using Generalised Estimation Equation analysis to determine the best predictors for each outcome over time. Predictors of work-related stress (patient care, staff issues, supervision/management issues, overtime and job demands) were entered into models with facets of burnout (emotional exhaustion, depersonalisation and personal accomplishment), job satisfaction (pay, promotion, supervision, fringe benefits, operating conditions, contingent rewards, co-workers, nature of work and communication) and general health (somatic symptoms, anxiety and insomnia, social dysfunction and severe depression) as outcomes. Facets of burnout were also entered as predictors into models with facets of job and general health as outcomes. Facets of job satisfaction were entered as predictors with facets of burnout and general health as outcomes. Odds Ratios (OR) were calculated as EXP (regression coefficient) and indicated the odds of predictors being associated with outcomes over time.

2.5 Ethical considerations

Ethics approval was obtained from Monash University Human Research Ethics Committee (MUHREC), Human Sciences Research Council (HSRC) and Gauteng's Department of Health (DoH). Informed consent was obtained from all participants in the study and anonymity was ensured through coding of data as well as presentation of aggregate findings in all publications.

3. Results

Tables 1–3 show the results of the GEE analysis [17].

DOI: http://dx.doi.org/10.5772/intechopen.89087

Work Related Stress Parameters	Burnout OR	Burnout 95% CI	Job Satisfaction OR	Job Satisfaction 95% CI	General Health OR	General Health 95% CI
Patient Care	2.24	1.94-2.59	2.63	1.35-5.16	2.50	1.32-4.73
Staff Issues	4.18	2.93-5.96	2.04	1.02-4.09	3.88	1.41-10.73
Job Demands	1.80	0.97-3.32	1.20	1.06-1.35	2.83	1.63-4.90
Lack of Support	4.37	2.89-6.62	1.70	1.41-2.03	1.83	1.33-2.53
Overtime	2.12	1.78-2.53	1.89	1.48-2.40	1.15	1.02-1.30

All stressors except job demands significantly predict burnout. All five stressors are significant predictors of job satisfaction and general health. Lack of support best predicts burnout over time, patient care best predicts job satisfaction over time and staff issues best predict general health over time.

Table 1.
GEE analysis of work-related stress as a predictor of burnout, job satisfaction and general health.

Burnout Parameters	Job Satisfaction OR	Job Satisfaction 95% CI	General Health OR	General Health 95% CI
Emotional Exhaustion	2.37	2.13-2.63	1.93	1.81-2.06
Depersonalisation	0.87	0.78-0.96	1.22	1.13-1.32
Personal Accomplishment	1.49	1.36-1.63	1.08	1.01-1.14

Emotional exhaustion is the most significant predictor of job satisfaction and general health.

Table 2.
GEE analysis of burnout as a predictor of job satisfaction and general health.

Job Satisfaction Parameters	Burnout OR	Burnout 95% CI	General Health OR	General Health 95% CI
Pay	1.07	0.99-1.15	0.91	0.84-0.99
Promotion	1.14	1.05-1.23	1.22	1.14-1.31
Supervision	1.10	0.98-1.23	0.93	0.86-1.01
Fringe Benefits	1.03	0.97-1.10	1.08	1.01-1.15
Operating Conditions	0.87	1.00-1.15	1.08	0.99-1.16
Contingent Rewards	0.95	0.89-1.01	0.99	0.93-1.06
Co-workers	0.95	0.88-1.03	0.70	0.64-0.76
Nature of Work	1.07	0.96-1.20	1.34	1.21-1.49
Communication	0.92	0.85-0.98	0.85	0.79-0.93

Job satisfaction with promotion is the most significant predictor of burnout and job satisfaction with nature of work is the most significant predictor of general health.

Table 3.
GEE analysis of job satisfaction as a predictor of burnout and general health.

4. Discussion

This study longitudinally examined work-related stress in relation to burnout, job satisfaction and general health among South African nurses. The findings of this study suggest that of all the five stressors contributing to work-related stress, job demands do not have an effect on burnout, lack of support is the most significant predictor of burnout among nurses, stress related to patient care most significantly predicts job satisfaction and stress related to staff issues best predicts general health. Although burnout and job satisfaction also predict general health of nurses, this study found that burnout is a better predictor. Emotional exhaustion best predicts general health over time but is a better predictor of job satisfaction. Burnout is also a better predictor of job satisfaction than vice versa [17].

The findings also confirmed that security risk in the workplace was the most influential work-related stressor associated with job satisfaction and general health of nurses at baseline. However, over time, lack of support, patient care and staff issues became more influential work-related stressors affecting burnout, job satisfaction and general health of nurses respectively. Although burnout predicts general health over time, it is a stronger predictor of job satisfaction. More specifically, it was found that, over time, lack of support leads to burnout among nurses and staff issues compromise the general health of nurses. Emotional exhaustion in particular is important in determining job satisfaction levels of nurses [17].

These findings differ a little from the previously proposed model based on existing literature (**Figure 1**), suggesting that work-related stressors including inadequate resources, lack of recognition and autonomy as well as peer relationships are associated with job satisfaction [18–20]. Lower job satisfaction is shown to have a direct negative effect on burnout among nurses [21, 22], which impacts general health outcomes [10]. These findings are supported by various theories including one of the first occupational stress theories namely the role stress model, which suggests that stressful role expectations compromise job satisfaction, exhaust physical energy and result in poor health outcomes [23]. Similarly, process models such as Kahn and Byosiere's causal stress theory posits that stressors are associated with responses (job satisfaction) and consequences (burnout and illness) [24].

Despite empirical support for existing frameworks, it is important to note that these largely examine relationships between variables with less focus on the processes through which the variables interact with each other. For example, Karasek's demands-control model posits that high strain situations (high demands and low control) increase the likelihood of poor health outcomes (heart disease and depression) [25]. However, this view does not account for internal processes including appraisal of stressors affecting various outcomes. This is important given that stress is a subjective experience that may affect outcomes differentially. Siegrist's effort-reward imbalance model is one of the few contemporary models that considers the role of environmental influences and individual perceptions [26]. However, some researchers have alluded to the idea that the consideration of individual differences and internal processes are limited to intrinsic factors [27].

Modern work places are affected by multiple stressors that are dynamic in nature. These have the potential to affect a number of outcomes. However, existing stress models do not explore a multitude of independent variables affecting several outcomes. For example, Hackman and Oldham's theory focusing on the impact of job characteristics (task identity, task significant, autonomy) on outcomes (satisfaction, absenteeism) includes examination of a limited number of characteristics and outcomes [28]. This theory seems to limit the explanatory power of independent variables and their effect on a number of outcomes.

More recent stress models such as demand skill support model [29] also focus on a few factors affecting stress in multiple settings. This theory is based on the presumption that the effect of stressful work environments are similar across individuals and occupations, which prevents an in depth understanding of stress and its outcomes for individuals in different contexts with different characteristics [27]. A recent study showing that personal stress is a better predictor of burnout and general health than job satisfaction, which is better predicted by work stress, confirms this assertion [30].

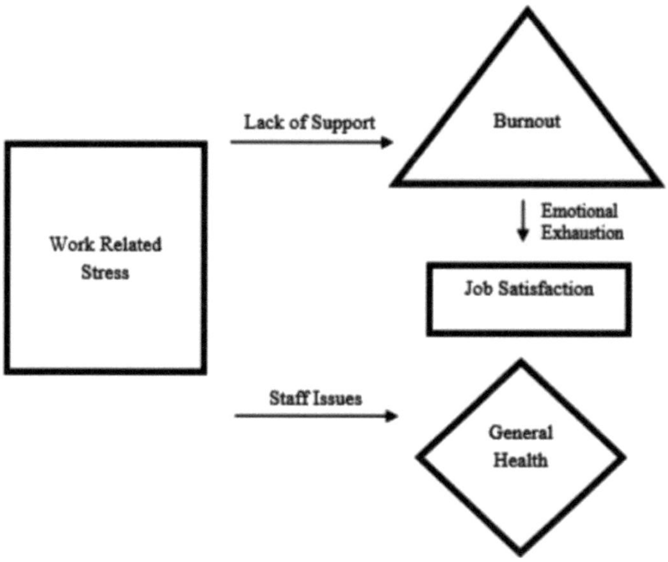

Figure 2.
Proposed model illustrating the relationships between work-related stress, burnout, job satisfaction and general health over time.

Based on some of the shortcomings of existing theoretical models, a revised model reflecting the findings of this study is proposed in **Figure 2**.

Contrary to the existing model (**Figure 1**), the proposed model suggests that work-related stress is associated with job satisfaction through burnout. In differing from the previous model, this model also suggests that burnout leads to lower job satisfaction rather than vice versa. Although burnout is associated with general health of nurses, this model indicates a stronger relationship between stress related to staff issues and poor general health outcomes for nurses [17].

This model incorporates appraisal and perception of stressors that affect burnout, job satisfaction and general health. Examination of the frequency and severity of stressors controls for the over-estimation of effects resulting from rare but highly stressful situations, while underestimating the effects of moderate but frequently occurring stressful situations [12]. This is important in determining whether stress is experienced considering that stressors may not contribute to stress unless they are perceived as such [31].

This model focuses on specific aspects of stress and burnout that affect job satisfaction and general health outcomes. Simultaneous examination of a multitude of contributing factors and outcomes provides an improved understanding of the complex processes through which stress affects burnout, job satisfaction and general health. This indicates a diversion from the one size fits all approach of several stress models in that it focuses specifically on how stressors contributing to stress among South African nurses affect burnout, job satisfaction and general health. It is important to know what stressful experiences are like for nurses working in difficult conditions, as well as the outcomes that are associated with this. This knowledge could inform the design of relevant interventions that are suitable to this population and other similar populations.

A key strength of this study is that it provides empirical evidence for relationships between work-related stress, burnout, job satisfaction and general health of nurses over time. Contribution of context specific findings, including the role of security risks in predicting job satisfaction and general health among South African nurses provides a foundation for further research examining work-related stress, burnout, job satisfaction and general health of nurses in other South African provinces as well as other developing countries. Furthermore, the proposed model could be used as a foundation for further research exploring mediating/moderating roles of burnout and job satisfaction.

Existing policies and practices appear to discard the issue of difficult working environments in developing countries, whereby policy related to health workforce wellbeing is not prioritized and mostly lacking [32]. This is apparent in the South African context given the current strategic plan for health practice, which is heavily based on anecdotal evidence owing to limited empirical evidence [1]. McInerney and Suleman confirm that one of the major barriers in implementing evidence based practice in South Africa is insufficient evidence [33]. This lack of evidence prevents application of findings to other developing countries where limited research also prevents evidence based practice [34]. It is clear that such gaps in policy and practice are due to limited evidence focusing on working conditions among health workers in developing countries. Evidence based practice involves the use of evidence to support decision making processes within healthcare systems [35]. This requires broader application of many forms of evidence including empirical studies and reviews, thereby ensuring comprehensive research utilisation. This need for evidence emphasizes the importance of this study in providing strong empirical evidence to inform human resources for health policy and practice in developing countries.

Considering the findings of this study, the following strategies are recommended for addressing work-related stress, burnout, job satisfaction and general health of nurses in South Africa and other developing countries:

- Improving security for nurses in their working environment while promoting job satisfaction and general health of nurses. Such improvements can be achieved through increased presence of security personnel and training on violence prevention as well as aggressive behavior management. The WHO's framework for addressing security risks in the workplace suggests ensuring safe access to and from the workplace as well as installing alarm systems and surveillance cameras [36]. It is also important that the risks be assessed and mitigated in light of organisational context when creating safe work environments [37]. These interventions could be applied within South African hospitals following evaluation of their feasibility and effectiveness within this context.

- Support from supervisors and colleagues to reduce the impact of burnout on physical and mental health of nurses. This support can be achieved through various strategies involving recognition for good work as well as staff support programs focusing on counseling and career advancement [38]. Evaluation of these strategies within developing contexts is necessary to ensure effectiveness.

- Creating supportive environments to improve job performance and encourage a sense of personal accomplishment as well as job satisfaction. This can be achieved through availability of adequate resources as well as healthy relationships between supervisors and colleagues [38, 39].

Implementation of these would require a multi-sectoral approach involving the government, department of health, academic leaders and researchers, nursing associations, healthcare providers, non-governmental organisations and nurses themselves. This array of stakeholders with a range of aims, capabilities and interests will facilitate an interactive approach for conversion of recommendations to policy and practice [40].

5. Conclusion

This chapter offers a better understanding of relationships between work-related stress, burnout, job satisfaction and general health of nurses. Over time, burnout plays a more important role in influencing job satisfaction among nurses. Interventions aimed at improving job satisfaction among nurses may reduce the negative impact of burnout on nurses' health, thereby encouraging quality nursing practice and patient outcomes. Policies and practices aimed at reducing work-related stress and burnout, while improving job satisfaction and general health of nurses, should be informed by this knowledge.

Acknowledgements

Sincere thanks to Professor Brian Oldenburg, Professor Karl Peltzer and Professor Dragan Ilic for their contribution to this study. A special thanks to the hospital management teams and nurse participants without whom this study would not have been possible.

Author details

Natasha Khamisa
IIE MSA, Johannesburg, South Africa

*Address all correspondence to: nkhamisa@iie.msa.co.za

References

[1] Department of Health. Strategic plan for nurse education, training and practice 2012/13-2016/17. Available from: http://www.sanc.co.za/archive/archive2013/NursingStrategy2013.html [Accessed: 30 June 2019]

[2] South African Nursing Council. Distribution of nursing manpower vs population in South Africa. Available from: http://www.sanc.co.za/stats/stat2017/Year%202017%20Provincial%20Distribution%20Stats.pdf [Accessed: 30 June 2019]

[3] Jordan TR, Khubchandani J, Wiblishauser M. The impact of perceived stress and coping adequacy on the health of nurses: A pilot investigation. Nursing Research & Practice. 2016;**2016**:1-11. DOI: 10.1155/2016/5843256

[4] Aiken LH, Sermeus W, Van den Heede K, Sloane DM, Busse R, McKee M, et al. Patient safety, satisfaction, and quality of hospital care: Cross sectional surveys of nurses and patients in 12 countries in Europe and the United States. BMJ. 2012;**344**:1-14. DOI: 10.1136/bmj.e1717

[5] Sherwood G, Barnsteiner J, editors. Quality and Safety in Nursing: A Competency Approach to Improving Outcomes. 2nd ed. New Jersey: John Wiley & Sons; 2017. 5 p

[6] Freudenberger HJ. Staff burn-out. Journal of Social Issues. 1974;**30**:159-165. DOI: 10.1111/j.1540-4560.1974.tb00706.x

[7] Maslach C. Burnout: The Cost of Caring. New Jersey: Prentice-Hall; 2006. 192 p. DOI. 10.1176/ps.34.7.650

[8] Maslach C, Schaufeli WB, Leiter MP. Job burnout. Annual Review of Psychology. 2001;**52**:397-422. DOI: 10.1146/annurev.psych.52.1.397

[9] Cooper CL, Dewe PJ, O'Driscoll MP. Organizational Stress: A Review and Critique of Theory, Research, and Applications. Thousand Oaks: Sage; 2001. 282 p. DOI: 10.4135/9781452231235

[10] Dugani S, Afari H, Hirschhorn LR, Ratcliffe H, Veillard J, Martin G, et al. Prevalence and factors associated with burnout among frontline primary health care providers in low and middle income countries: A systematic review. Gates Open Research. 2018;**2**:4. DOI: 10.12688/gatesopenres.12779.3

[11] Rothmann S, van der Colff JJ, Rothmann JC. Occupational stress of nurses in South Africa. Curationis. 2006;**29**:24-25. DOI: 10.4102/curationis.v29i2.1069

[12] Spielberger CD, Vagg PR, Wasala CF. Occupational stress: Job pressures and lack of support. In: Quick JC, Tetrick LE, editors. Handbook of Occupational Health Psychology. Washington: American Psychological Association; 2003. pp. 185-200. DOI: 10.1037/10474-009

[13] Spector PE. Job Satisfaction: Application, Assessment, Causes and Consequences. London: Sage Publications; 1997

[14] Piko BF. Burnout, role conflict, job satisfaction and psychosocial health among Hungarian health care staff: A questionnaire survey. International Journal of Nursing Studies. 2006;**43**:311-318. DOI: 10.1016/j.ijnurstu.2005.05.003

[15] Khamisa N, Peltzer K, Oldenburg B. Burnout in relation to specific contributing factors and health outcomes among nurses: A systematic review. International Journal of Environmental Research and Public Health. 2013;**10**:2214-2240. DOI: 10.3390/ijerph10062214

[16] Jamal M, Baba VV. Job stress and burnout among Canadian managers and nurses: An empirical examination. Canadian Journal of Public Health. 2000;**91**:454-458. DOI: 10.1007/BF03404828

[17] Khamisa N, Peltzer K, Ilic D, Oldenburg B. Work related stress, burnout, job satisfaction and general health of nurses: A follow up study. International Journal of Nursing Practice. 2016;**22**:538-545. DOI: 10.1111/ijn.12455

[18] Djukic M, Kovner C, Budin WC, Norman R. Physical work environment: Testing an expanded model of job satisfaction in a sample of registered nurses. Nursing Research. 2010;**59**:441-451. DOI: 10.1097/NNR.0b013e3181fb2f25

[19] Tourangeau AE, Patterson E, Saari M, Thomson H, Cranley L. Work-related factors influencing home care nurse intent to remain employed. Health Care Management Review. 2017;**42**:87-97. DOI: 10.1097/HMR.0000000000000093

[20] Halcomb E, Smyth E, McInnes S. Job satisfaction and career intentions of registered nurses in primary health care: An integrative review. BMC Family Practice. 2018;**19**:136. DOI: 10.1186/s12875-018-0819-1

[21] Fennessey AG. The relationship of burnout, work environment, and knowledge to self-reported performance of physical assessment by registered nurses. Medical-Surgical Nursing. 2016;**25**:346

[22] Whitebird RR, Solberg LI, Crain AL, Rossom RC, Beck A, Neely C, et al. Clinician burnout and satisfaction with resources in caring for complex patients. General Hospital Psychiatry. 2017;**44**:91-95. DOI: 10.1016/j.genhosppsych.2016.03.004

[23] Kahn RL, Wolfe DM, Quinn RP, Snoek JD. Organizational Stress: Studies in Role Conflict and Ambiguity. New York: Wiley; 1964

[24] Kahn RL, Byosiere P. Stress in organisations: Overview, reflection and evaluation of the Kahn-Byosiere model. International Journal of Psychology. 2004;**39**:503

[25] Karasek R. Job demands, job decision latitude and mental strain: Implications for job redesign. Administrative Science Quarterly. 1979;**24**:285-306. DOI: 10.2307/2392498

[26] Siegrist J. Adverse health effects of high-effort/low-reward conditions. Journal of Occupational Health Psychology. 2006;**1**:27-41. DOI: 10.1037/1076-8998.1.1.27

[27] Mark GM, Smith AP. Stress models: A review and suggested new direction. In: Houdmont J, Leka S, editors. Occupational Health Psychology. Nottingham: Nottingham University Press; 2008. pp. 111-144

[28] Hackman JR, Oldham GR. Work Redesign. Massachusetts: Addison-Wesley; 1980

[29] Van Veldhoven M, Taris TW, De Jonge J, Broersen S. The relationship between work characteristics and employee health and well-being: How much complexity do we really need? International Journal of Stress Management. 2005;**12**:3-28. DOI: 10.1037/1072-5245.12.1.3

[30] Khamisa N, Peltzer K, Ilic D, Oldenburg B. Effect of personal and work stress on burnout, job satisfaction and general health of hospital nurses in South Africa. Health SA Gesondheid. 2017;**22**:252-258. DOI: 10.4102/hsag.v22i0.1011

[31] Briner RB, Harris C, Daniels K. How do work stress and coping work? Toward a fundamental theoretical reappraisal. British Journal of Guidance

and Counselling. 2004;**32**:223-234. DOI: 10.1080/03069880410001692256

[32] Hornung S, Rousseau DM, Glaser J, Angerer P, Weigl M. Beyond top-down and bottom-up work redesign: Customizing job content through idiosyncratic deals. Journal of Organizational Behavior. 2010;**31**: 187-215. DOI: 10.1002/job.625

[33] Mclnerney P, Suleman F. Exploring knowledge, attitudes, and barriers toward the use of evidence-based practice amongst academic health care practitioners in their teaching in a south African university: A pilot study. Worldviews on Evidence-Based Nursing. 2010;7:90-97. DOI: 10.1111/j.1741-6787.2009.00180.x

[34] Majid S, Foo S, Luyt B, Zhang X, Theng YL, Chang YK, et al. Adopting evidence-based practice in clinical decision making: Nurses' perceptions, knowledge, and barriers. Journal of the Medical Library Association. 2011;**99**:229

[35] Gordon HJ, Demerouti E, Le Blanc PM, Bakker AB, Bipp T, Verhagen MA. Individual job redesign: Job crafting interventions in healthcare. Journal of Vocational Behavior. 2018;**104**:98-114. DOI: 10.1016/j.jvb.2017.07.002

[36] World Health Organization. Framework guidelines for addressing workplace violence in the health sector. Available from: http://www.who.int/violence_injury_prevention/violence/activities/workplace/en/ [Accessed on 02 July 2019]

[37] Wressell JA, Rasmussen B, Driscoll A. Exploring the workplace violence risk profile for remote area nurses and the impact of organisational culture and risk management strategy. Collegian. 2018;**25**:601-606. DOI: 10.1016/j.colegn.2018.10.005

[38] Kutney-Lee A, Wu ES, Sloane DM, Aiken LH. Changes in hospital nurse work environments and nurse job outcomes: An analysis of panel data. International Journal of Nursing Studies. 2013;**50**:195-201. DOI: 10.1016/j.ijnurstu.2012.07.014

[39] Ulrich B, Barden C, Cassidy L, Varn-Davis N. Critical care nurse work environments 2018: Findings and implications. Critical Care Nurse. 2019;**39**:67-84. DOI: 10.4037/ccn2019605

[40] Cho H, Han K. Associations among nursing work environment and health-promoting behaviors of nurses and nursing performance quality: A multilevel modeling approach. Journal of Nursing Scholarship. 2018;**50**: 403-410. DOI: 10.1111/jnu.12390